Mom Fell, Now What?
Field Notes from the Front Line of Caregiving

Mom Fell, Now What?

FIELD NOTES
FROM THE FRONT LINE
OF CAREGIVING

KATHLEEN RAWLINGS

Mom Fell, Now What?
Field Notes from the Front Line of Caregiving

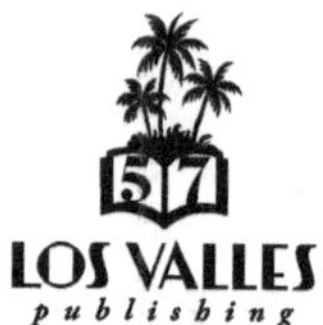

Cover Design by Alan Pranke
Paperback ISBN: 979-8-9935244-0-5
eBook ISBN: 979-8-9935244-1-2
Audiobook ISBN: 979-8-9935244-2-9

Scan to visit: **momfell-nowwhat.com** →

First Edition 2026
PRINTED IN THE UNITED STATES OF AMERICA

Table of Contents

Introduction

If you're reading this book, you've likely gotten *the call* in some form or another. An aging loved one needs help.

When I got *the call,* I was thrust into an adrenaline-fueled panic. I couldn't get to St. Louis fast enough. A few months ago, I was schlepping up the stairs of my son's dorm on move-in day, stocking shelves with oversized boxes of Cheez-Its, and feeling a little (a lot) sad about him leaving home. Now I'm feverishly trying to catch a plane to get to Mom before she dies and wondering. *How does this happen?*

I'm finally finding my stride again, rediscovering myself as a fifty-*something*-year-old. Things are moving at a calm, predictable pace. My husband and I aren't empty nesters–yet–but we are halfway there. One son is in high school, and the other is away at college. I cook less chicken, buy less toilet paper, and fold less laundry. I like the idea of getting reacquainted with my husband. BC (before children) we used to go to the gym together, and we've just started doing this again. It's nice. We are reconnecting. On Saturday evening, we have date night. We cap off the week with pizza and a glass of wine at a neighborhood bistro. Sure, I still worry about the kids, but I worry less. With them out of sight, I focus less on them and more on me.

But all this is about to change. I'm being called back home. Home (to a city I left over twenty years ago) to care for an aging parent.

One in every four adults is a caregiver.

Caregivers are diverse across race, income, and generation. And, twenty-nine percent are sandwich generation caregivers, meaning they are supporting both children and older adults. According to Jonathan Vespa, a senior demographer for the U.S. Census Bureau, our nation is heading toward a "gray tsunami."

Like most people, I never imagined I'd be swept up in this "tsunami." Sure, the news is full of political debates about our aging population, but I tune it out. It feels distant, irrelevant. Not my problem.

Terms like *skilled rehab, activities of daily living,* and *Medicare supplements* are phrases without meaning. I have no context, and frankly, no interest. These are things my parents worry about, not me.

Until everything changed—the day I got *the call.*

> By 2040, 21 percent of the U.S. population will be sixty-five and older, up from sixteen percent in 2019. In twenty years, we will have over seventy-seven million older Americans. There will be more elderly people than children under eighteen. According to a *Caregiving* in the U.S 2025 report, sixty-three million Americans will be caregivers, a nearly 50 percent increase since 2015.

Looking back, I probably had an inkling of what was coming, but I didn't want to face it. I remember a phone call with my sister shortly before Dad passed. I was sitting in my car, about to head into a local takeout spot. We chatted about the usual—kids, work and our parents. Then Dad's declining health came up.

I thanked her for taking care of our parents. She still lives in St. Louis. I live in Texas. We exchanged a few more pleasantries, and then she said something that stopped me cold. She said, "I'll take care of Dad. Mom is yours."

Mom is mine? Wait—what? No. How can I take care of Mom? I don't even live in the same city. Dad's the one with heart issues and diabetes. Mom's physical health is fine, aside from her chronic high blood pressure. Her challenge is mental health. She's a ball of stress fighting anxiety, phobias and mood swings. *She's also obstinate, ornery, and impossible. Nope. I'm not taking this on. I'll just pretend that nothing is going to change.*

If you've had a moment like this where you see the inevitable coming but can't bring yourself to prepare for it, don't beat yourself up. There's no shame in denial. It works perfectly, until it doesn't. And if you're holding this book, chances are denial is no longer working for you.

When I got the call that Mom had fallen and had been on the floor for four days, I had no idea I was about to be swept into a tidal wave of change. Booking a flight and rushing to her bedside was just the beginning.

My first thought: *Where do I begin? I don't know what I don't know.* There's no plan, not for me, and certainly not for Mom, and I am part of a generation that is independent, gritty and decisive. We work hard. We play hard. We expect the best, prepare for the worst, and we always— *always*—have a backup plan. So, when caregiving lands in our laps, we don't crumble. We adapt. We research. We organize, and we lead.

No Plan Is Not an Option

Whether living across town or across the country, caring for an aging loved one is hard. There's no gentle onboarding and no gradual ramp-up. One day, I'm living my adult life and the next, I'm auto enrolled into a crash course on caregiving, learning a language I have never spoken, partaking in a subculture I never knew existed and assuming a role I never asked for or wanted. In an instant, I'm a member of Mom's care team. It's like becoming a parent for the first time, only in reverse. And until now, no instruction manual existed. This book is about to change that.

Chapter Structure

To support you along your journey, I'm sharing lessons learned, hard-won insights and best practices, offered in bite-sized chunks. This isn't a physics book. You don't have to master one chapter before moving on to the next. It's a just-in-time reference filled with relatable, practical advice to help make sense of terms like Activities of Daily Living (ADL), Medicare Part A, aging in place, and the difference between assisted living and skilled nursing.

The chapters contain resources, tips, questions to ask and things to consider. Feel free to skip around. Take what you need, when you need it, and leave the rest. One thing to consider, I recommend reading not only the chapter about your current situation but also the one that follows. It might just prepare you for what's around the corner. Each chapter is designed to meet you where you are—with clarity, empathy, and practical support. Inside, you'll find:

- A personal story to set the stage and remind you that you're not alone

- Helpful tips and call-outs woven throughout the narrative

- Clear definitions of key terms and phrases

- Thoughtful questions to guide conversations and decisions

- Curated resources and tools for making the next step easier

Whether the relationship with your loved one is warm and close, or one marred by tension and complexity, stepping into a caregiving role can feel overwhelming. My hope for you is simple. I want you to know others have walked the path before you, and many are walking it beside you now. *Mom Fell, Now What? Field Notes from the Frontline of Caregiving* is here to offer comfort, support and guidance as you navigate the twists and turns of caregiving. May it help you feel more connected as you journey forward.

CHAPTER 1

The Call

It is Thanksgiving week, and I duck out of work early for some long-overdue mom-and-son time. My college freshman made the twelve-hour trek home, and I'm determined to soak up every moment with him. We are three frames into a casual game of bowling when my phone buzzes with the call that changes life as I know it.

It's my nephew. He's at my mother's house. He says, "I found Mardy (our family name for grandmother) on the floor. She's conscious, but I can't understand her. I called 911. The paramedics are on their way."

I freeze. My brain short-circuits. *Mom is on the floor?* I'm in Texas. She's in Missouri. This can't be happening. I can't process it. *Think. Respond. Say something—anything.*

In a moment, everything changes. One minute I'm carefree, enjoying time with my son and the next, I'm plunged headfirst into an unexpected role, caregiver for my aging mother.

I explain the situation to my son. We turn in our bowling shoes and race home. My mind floods with thoughts. *Can I even get a flight out? It's Thanksgiving. It's going to cost a fortune. Is she dying? Is she already dead?*

Should I pack for a funeral?

How can two little words–Mom fell–stop me in my tracks? I'll tell you how: while we were busy vying for the next promotion or shuttling our kids to baseball games and dance recitals, our parents were aging. Since I am still raising my own kids, the idea of caring for an aging parent is the last thing on my mind. And yet here I am, an official inductee of the sandwich generation. I feel like a panini–grilled, flattened, and slightly burnt.

I toss clothes and toiletries into a bag, call my husband, text my other son, and reach out to my sister. I ask her to pick me up at the airport when I arrive. The essentials are covered. Everyone knows. Then it hits me: work. I send my boss a quick text:

My mom is in the hospital, and I'm flying to St. Louis tonight. I'll check in tomorrow.

The message is brief, direct, and all I can manage in the moment.

Once at the airport, I board the plane and settle in. We wait for our turn to take off. Eventually, we are wheels up ascending to our cruising altitude. Time is crawling. This hour-and-a-half flight feels like a transatlantic haul. When family is in crisis, every minute drags like a treadmill cranked to a level-ten incline. I glance at my watch; stare out the window, and glance down again. Time doesn't budge. I shift in my seat and try to quiet my mind. The night sky is stunning—clear and still. I pray. *Heavenly Father, please let Mom be okay. Watch over her. Keep her safe.*

My neck tightens. Anxiety climbs. My heart races. Saliva pools in my mouth. No time for tears. Not now. There's too much to do. I whisper another prayer under my breath, hoping to slow my pulse. Another glance at my wrist. *The numbers on my watch numbers aren't changing.* Time is frozen.

Then finally, the captain's voice: "Flight attendants, prepare for landing."

The plane touches down and taxis to the gate. The cabin lights barely flicker on, and I'm on my feet. We deplane, and somewhere between a walk and a jog, I rush down the concourse. I make my way to the exit, and the sliding doors squeak open. Cold November air slaps my cheeks. Instantly, my eyes water.

I spot my sister, toss my bag in the back of her car and slide into the passenger seat. "How is she? Is she conscious? What do we know?" I don't even pause to hear a response. I just continue peppering my sister with questions.

"I was at the hospital just before I came to get you. I don't know much yet. I met the ambulance at the ER. Matthew found her. The last time I talked to her was last Wednesday," Tina says.

It's Tuesday. Neither of us has spoken to Mom in almost a week. I usually call on Sundays, but I skipped this week. I remember a nagging instinct telling me to call, and I ignored it. *If I had called, we could have checked on her sooner.*

My sister and I ride in silence. The short drive to the hospital feels like an eternity. *This can't be the fastest route.* Fear is mounting and my thoughts are spiraling.

Eventually, we pull up to a modest, four-story hospital—not a trauma center, just the closest one to Mom's house. I jump out, speed past Tina, slip through the sliding doors and head straight to the elevators. We step inside. I stare at the panel of buttons. "What floor?" I ask. Tina reaches over and presses four. "She's in room 415," she says. The elevator starts moving. We ride in silence.

When the doors open, I am the first one out. I see the sign on the wall 410 – 420, and head down the hallway scanning room numbers. I approach 415. It is across from the nurses' station. The door is half-closed. I nudge it open and step in.

The TV is on but muted. The room is quiet except for the steady chirping of the monitor beside her bed. Between the beeps, I hear the soft hiss of oxygen filling the tubes under Mom's nose. *Why is she on oxygen?* This all feels surreal. I'm not ready for this—not emotionally, not mentally.

I move toward the bed. "Hi, Mom. How are you?"

"Who's there?" she asks, her voice thin and raspy. She's dehydrated and weak.

She doesn't turn her head, just stares at the ceiling.

What does she mean, 'Who's there?' She only has two daughters and Tina met her at the ER.

"It's me. Kathy."

"Kathy?" she repeats puzzled.

Then her expression changes.

"Oh, good. I'm glad you're here," she says.

"Do you see the Christmas present over there? That red box? Can you move it so they don't take it?" She's pointing at the red hazmat box attached to the wall. Tina and I exchange glances. Tina leans in and whispers.

"She's been without fluids for four days. The human body can only go three days without water," Tina says, her voice sounding clinical. "Her dementia has been progressing. She's experiencing diminished mental capacity."

Wait. What? I can't absorb all of this. Tina's reciting survival stats, Mom is mistaking the medical waste bin for a pile of Christmas gifts, and now I'm learning she's hallucinating because of dementia.

Slow down. One step at a time.

Mom continues mumbling nonsense until she talks herself to sleep.

I glance at the whiteboard beneath the TV. Written in green marker:

Nurse—Beth; Tech—Jayme; Daughter—Tina

Tina's phone number is listed below.

I know that Tina lives here and I don't, but I can't help but feel a twinge of jealousy. We are both points of contact. It's not that Mom doesn't acknowledge me—it's that the hospital team does not. And this moment becomes a preview of what's to come.

All the correct forms are on file. I'm authorized to receive all the medical and financial information about her. But in the world of caregiving, presence often trumps paperwork.

> HIPAA stands for the Health Insurance Portability and Accountability Act, a U.S. federal law that protects the privacy and security of individuals' medical information and sets standards for electronic health records.
>
> HIPAA
> - Limits who can access and share a patient's health information
>
> - Requires safeguards for electronic health records (EHRs)

- Ensures people can maintain health insurance coverage when changing jobs

- Establishes penalties for misuse or unauthorized disclosure of health data

Maybe it's the close-knit, no one-moves-away-from-St. Louis mindset. Maybe it's just whoever fills out the intake form. Either way, as I repeatedly experience over the days, weeks, and years to come, Tina gets the first call. I get the second, if I get one at all. No matter how many times I reassure the staff that Tina and I communicate everything, they still default to her. I'm always playing catch-up. This isn't my sister's fault. It's just the way things are.

I walk over to the whiteboard, uncap the marker, and add my name and phone number. It's a small gesture, but it feels important—like claiming a place in Mom's care narrative.

Coordinating patient care within the tangled web of the healthcare system is no small feat. With countless moving parts and layers of communication, challenges are inevitable. Whether you live across the country or just a few miles away, navigating the healthcare landscape requires sharp communication skills and unwavering follow-through.

Nurse Beth appears in the doorway. Tina and I step out of the room and into the hallway. With my anxiety still in overdrive, I drill Beth with questions rambling them off one after the other, barely pausing to breathe. My intensity isn't landing. Beth is reserved and distant, clearly eager to cut the conversation short. Finally, she offers, "Just come early tomorrow. You should be able to find out more then. If you're here most of the day, you'll catch the house doc and the specialists as they come through."

I force a polite smile and thank her.

Tina and I head toward the elevators.

"I guess I'll get here around six in the morning," I say.

The drive to Mom's house is quiet. I thank Tina for picking me up, grab my luggage from the back, punch in the garage code, and step inside.

The house feels familiar—but different. Everything has changed.

CHAPTER 2

The Hospital Stay

Topics

— When Memory Meets Loss: Talking About Deceased
Loved Ones with Dementia Patients

— Falls and Aging: What the Data Reveals

— Teamwork in Triage: Asking Questions
and Being Present

— Strategic Timing: Why Rounds Matter
in Patient Advocacy

— Getting Organized and Keeping Good Notes

The alarm buzzes—5:30 a.m. Even though my eyes are closed, I'm not really sleeping. Between worrying about Mom and trying to settle into the forty-year-old rock-hard mattress (the most comfortable bed in her house), I spent the night in a state of restless limbo. It's like sleeping on an airplane: eyes closed, body still, but nothing restful about it. This is the beginning of acclimating to what will become my new normal—life at Mom's house.

I turn off the alarm, roll out of bed, shower, and dry my hair. Everything about this setup is uncomfortable. Threadbare bath towels, a garage-sale hairdryer with one setting, and one-ply toilet paper. *Who buys one-ply?*

It's barely a step above sandpaper. Mental note: pick up toilet paper on the way home. By the time I'm dressed and ready, I've got fifteen minutes to get to the hospital if I want to catch the doctors during rounds and hear the latest updates.

I open the refrigerator and hunt for an unopened bottle of water, a rare luxury in a house where everything gets reused at least twice. No luck. Shifting gears, I realize I left home without a notepad; I open a desk drawer in search of a legal pad. No legal pad in sight but tucked among the clutter is my eighth-grade Shawn Cassidy Trapper Keeper and a half-used Powerpuff Girls spiral notebook. Not exactly professional, but it'll do. I grab the notebook and head out the door.

When Memory Meets Loss: Talking About Deceased Loved Ones with Dementia Patients

I ease into Mom's hospital room, sidestepping the half-drawn privacy curtain and the bedside table. I can't tell whether she slept well or was awake all night. No nurse or tech in sight yet. On the tray are a half-eaten graham cracker and a mini can of Sprite, small signs that she had a snack after I left.

I make my way over to the window, quietly setting down my computer bag. *So, this is my new remote office.* No Starbucks. No sit-stand desk, and no ergonomic chair. Instead, I make myself at home with vending-machine coffee, a vinyl recliner built for durability, not comfort, and a spotty unsecured Wi-Fi signal. The soundtrack has changed, too. Instead of yesterday's smooth jazz, I'm serenaded with Doris Day belting out "Que Sera Sera" on the hospital TV.

Mom is sleeping soundly; her breathing is raspy and labored. The room is still. It's the perfect time to catch up on emails, but the impulse to work feels distant. Instead, the urge to simply sit and watch her breathe takes over. The internal debate begins. *I'm being unproductive. I need to get my laptop out. I need to be working.* But something about the rise and fall of her chest, the soft rhythm of the monitor's beep, is cathartic.

After a while, Mom opens her eyes and says, "Oh, hi Kath. How long have you been here?"

I smile. "Not long. How are you feeling?"

"I'm thirsty," she says. "And I hurt all over."

"I'm sure you're sore, and I'm glad you're thirsty."

We're off to a better start than last night. She knows my name, and she's no longer mistaking the hazmat dispenser for a Christmas present. Holding the Styrofoam cup just below her chin, I bend the straw and she draws in the clear liquid.

"Is that Doris Day?" she asks.

"Yes."

After a short pause she says, "Do you see that woman over there on that bicycle? She keeps riding around the campground, and she's got those silly fringes hanging off the handlebars. That's my mom. Always showing off."

She's hallucinating again. Yesterday it was stolen Christmas gifts. Today, it's her mother, gone eight years now, riding a bike.

What's the right move here? Play along? Gently correct her? I decide to let her stay in the moment a little longer, then try to redirect her. "What's the name of this movie? Do you remember?" She is quiet again, but her gaze doesn't change. She continues staring out the window, lost in something I cannot see.

Minutes pass. She begins talking again, but the topic shifts. She asks, "Where's Joe? I don't understand why he won't come see me." She's talking about my father, who has been gone for three years. The question lands hard.

She turns toward me; her glossy green eyes search mine. "Where is he?" she insists.

Not sure if I tell her the truth or play along, I hesitate, then answer softly, "Mom, he can't come. He's no longer here."

Confusion floods her face. "What do you mean he's not here? Where is he?" Her voice trembles. I hold her gaze and feel my own eyes fill with tears. She's scared. Disoriented. "What do you mean? Is he…," she pauses, "dead?"

I look away.

"No!" she moans with agony. The grief is fresh, raw. Just as piercing as the day he died. Her pain is real. And so is mine. *Did I do the right thing?*

The answer isn't simple. It depends. Most dementia experts lean toward honesty, especially when the person is lucid enough to ask. But in moments like this, there's no perfect script. Only the hope that compassion, however imperfect, will carry through.

> Determining if a cognitively impaired person should be told about their spouse's death is a difficult decision. Experts suggest:
>
> - Telling the person at a time of day that is best for them
>
> - Making sure the place is free of distractions
>
> - Establishing the context: "I have some sad news about your brother Jack." Don't make it like a quiz: "Do you remember Jack?" Instead, help make clear whom you're talking about
>
> - It's okay to show emotion yourself. Take the person's hand
>
> *"Resource: Minimizing Grief for a Surviving Spouse with Dementia"* (https://www.agingcare.com)

As heartbreaking as it is to watch Mom relearn that Dad has died, something changes. It feels like a turning point, as if she's beginning to grasp the edges of her own confusion. Over the next several hours, we share stories.

She asks a flurry of questions. "How long have you been married? When did I stop working? How old are my grandsons? What grades are they in?"

Mom is beginning to act more like herself. It feels as though the fog is lifting, as she's starting to distinguish between distant memories and present day.

Falls and Aging: What the Data Reveals

The days blur together as I keep vigil at Mom's bedside. Time is distorted. Hours slip by like minutes, and days collapse into hours. She has been in the hospital for four days now, unable to get out of bed. Each attempt to move her ends in sharp, unbearable pain.

Eventually, an X-ray is ordered. A portable machine is wheeled in, and the technician snaps an image of her hip. It's confirmed. She has a fractured left hip. She's going to need surgery. Looks like my makeshift "remote office" at the hospital will be my work-from-home location for a while longer.

> According to *Falls and the Elderly by George F. Fuller,* patients rarely suffer just one fall. "A single fall is not always a sign of a major problem and an increased risk for subsequent falls. The fall may simply be an isolated event. However, recurrent falls, defined as more than two falls in a six-month period, should be evaluated for treatable causes. An immediate evaluation is required for falls that produce injuries or are associated with a new acute illness, loss of consciousness, fever or abnormal blood pressure."
>
> Source: Falls in the Elderly | AAFP

Under normal circumstances, a fractured hip might have been diagnosed earlier. But in Mom's case, the immediate priorities at admission were stabilizing her oxygen levels, getting her fluid levels up and ruling out major organ damage.

Teamwork in Triage: Asking Questions and Being Present

As Mom's marathon of declining health begins, so does my new role as patient advocate. And instead of taking part in a company function like "bring your daughter to work day," I'm flipping the script and bringing my best leadership and communication skills to my new job—Project Manager of Mom's Life.

I begin by trying to connect with Mom's hospital doctors to discuss her case. Availability is everything. My time takes a back seat to theirs, and this reality is both frustrating and exhausting. I'm at the mercy of their schedules. But they have something I need—information. Updates, insights, and answers. So, I wait.

Taking turns at the hospital with family or friends helps ensure someone's always there when a physician or specialist makes their rounds. For solo caregivers, some days may feel like endurance challenges, spending long hours waiting, just to catch a few minutes with the medical team.

Arriving early at the hospital has its advantages, especially during shift change. This is when the overnight team hands off notes and updates to those coming on duty. Often, the briefing happens in Mom's room where I hear firsthand how she's doing. I can ask questions and get up-to-the-minute details like blood work results, scheduled tests and vital-sign readings.

Today, during shift changeover I learn there are orders for a neurological consult, a dietary consultation and a request for a social worker to visit. Mom has an orthopedic surgeon assigned. Her medical team is expanding.

Forming strong connections with nurses and technicians can make all the difference. They're the ones who have access to the chart, spend the most time with the patient, notice subtle shifts in behavior, and often have a clearer sense of what's happening behind the scenes. Kindness goes a long way. Being respectful can open doors to information about your loved one's care.

As the list of specialists grows, so does the need for communication and coordination. Although nurses may share chart insights, they seldom do so voluntarily. Being inquisitive pays off.

As a patient advocate, asking questions is an important skill. Probe for information, ask follow-up questions and dig deeper to understand what the answers mean. If blood was drawn or a specimen collected a few days prior, ask if the results are in and if they are normal or if there is anything out of the ordinary.

During the shift change briefing, I ask, "Do we know a day and time yet for when they'll operate on Mom's hip?"

"It looks like they are aiming for Monday or Tuesday. They are trying to work her in."

"Monday or Tuesday?" I gristle. "They don't know? Am I just supposed to sit around all weekend waiting for someone to give me details?"

Clearly annoyed with my tone, the night nurse looks over the top of her glasses and then back to the computer screen. "Oh, nobody really does much over the weekend. Just plan on being here early Monday morning."

And so, I wait. Again. At the mercy of someone else's timeline, with no clarity or direction.

This exchange is just one of many conversations I'll have with medical teams in the months and years ahead, each one testing my patience as I try to hold my tongue and avoid saying something I'll later regret.

Hours pass, and right on schedule at 10:00 a.m. a woman from the cafeteria arrives with Mom's lunch tray. She greets Mom and begins listing the items on the tray: turkey, mashed potatoes and carrots.

Mom barks back, "No. I ordered a hamburger, no cheese, and peaches."

The woman glances at a slip of paper, "It says here you are on a low-sodium, diabetic diet."

"I am not," Mom insists. "I'm not diabetic."

"Well, it looks like you'll need to talk to dietary. This is what I've got for you now. Do you want it or not?"

Mom sighs and reluctantly accepts the tray. She's not happy, and I don't blame her. This is yet another stellar example of miscommunication. I need to figure out who to talk with to get the restrictions lifted. She picks at her dry turkey and cold mashed potatoes when a new face enters the room, Dr. Riley, Mom's orthopedic surgeon.

Strategic Timing: Why Rounds Matter in Patient Advocacy

They exchange pleasantries, bonding over the doctor's Irish heritage. Mom launches into stories: how she's never broken a bone, how she loves working in the yard, how she made varsity volleyball as a freshman. Dr. Riley listens with genuine interest, commending her toughness and athleticism.

"I'll be performing a full hip replacement," she says. "I've done this procedure hundreds of times, and I'm confident yours will go well."

To explain the fracture, she offers a metaphor: the femoral head has separated from the acetabulum, like a Tootsie Pop where the candy ball has snapped off the stick. "The medical term is arthroplasty," she adds with a smile. "In case anyone asks."

She has an impeccable bedside manner, and building trust with Mom is more than half the battle. Dr. Riley confirms that surgery will be early Monday morning, with prep starting at 7:00 a.m. *Finally, a clear answer.* Moments like this define why I spend countless hours at the hospital. I have specifics about Mom's pending procedure, and I've met her surgeon. I can put a face with a name, a small but meaningful step in making a connection and building a relationship.

Before leaving the room, Dr. Riley offers one more update: physical therapy and occupational therapy will begin on Tuesday morning. "We want to get you up and moving as soon as possible."

Getting Organized and Keeping Good Notes

I feel better. There now is a plan and I can get things in order. First up, brief my sister on the details from the conversation with Dr. Riley, and update Mom's medical journal A resource we grow to rely on as the twists and turns of her health journey unfold.

Capture specific milestone events like surgery dates, type of surgery performed, and the doctor performing the procedure. Include details such as the doctor's office phone number and location. (Refer to Chapter 3 for medical journal details.)

With a clear path ahead, I can begin charting a path forward balancing the demands of my professional job with my project manager role on Mom's care team. Accepting that she'll be hospitalized for a while longer means I must start shaping my new normal. I need to map out when I can realistically get work done, when I'll be available to speak with her medical team; and, probably most daunting, how I'm going to navigate life living at Mom's house for the foreseeable future.

Helpful Tips

- **Stay familiar with names and roles on the medical team.** Learn when nurses and techs rotate shifts and make an effort to build rapport. These are the people who spend the most time with a loved one, and they often share valuable insights. Nurses, in particular, may scan the chart and explain when tests are ordered, medications are adjusted, or X-rays are scheduled. A little connection goes a long way in staying informed.

- **Find out when doctors and specialists make their rounds.** Timing matters; being present during doctors' rounds can provide firsthand updates and a chance to ask questions.

- **Choose battles wisely.** Stress affects everyone differently, and high-pressure situations can amplify tensions. A little courtesy, patience, and respect can go a long way in building trust with medical staff.

- **Advocate for loved ones but let them speak for themselves.** Providers want to hear directly from the patient when possible. Resist the urge to jump in too quickly; give the patient time and space to share their experience before stepping in to clarify or fill in gaps.

- **Expect long hours at the hospital.** Sometimes, just being present at the hospital increases the likelihood of connecting with specialists and gathering information.

- **Take breaks.** Step outside. Take a walk around the hospital grounds. Visit the chapel. Practice a few minutes of meditation. And do not forget to eat, grabbing lunch at a nearby restaurant where waitstaff service is provided can feel like a small luxury in the middle of a long day.

- **It is okay to step away**. Balancing caregiving with work and personal responsibilities is hard. Stepping away from the hospital when needed is not irresponsible; it is survival.

RESOURCES

Falls in the Elderly | AAFP (https://www.aafp.org)

Hip Replacement Surgery: How it Works, Recovery Time | HSS (https://www.hss.edu)

Ways to reduce risk of falling among the elderly - Bing video)

What Is a Hospitalist Doctor? What They Do, When to See One, and What to Expect (https://www.webmd.com)

CHAPTER 3

Project Manager of Mom's Life

Topics

— Two Journals: Keeping Up with Medical
and Financial Information

— Tracking Medical Details: Staying on Top of Allergies,
Medications, and Physicians

— Managing Financial Information: A Key Role
in Coordinated Care

— Demystifying the Living Trust: What It Is
and Why It Matters

What knowledge, skills and behaviors make a successful project manager? According to Coursera "A project manager (PM) manages people, tasks, schedules, and resources throughout the project lifecycle." And when I drop this same question into my favorite search engine or artificial intelligence (AI) tool, the description is clear: a PM must be organized, have great communication skills, demonstrate leadership, have technological proficiency, be adaptable and manage their time well. Exactly the skills I need as the project manager of Mom's life. The difference is that instead of earning a generous salary, I'm doing it for free. And as a bonus, I'm partnering with a sibling, a project requirement that demands diplomacy and compromise.

From the moment I'm thrust into my new role as a member of Mom's care team, I know that keeping good notes is critical. Whether it's tracking names, addresses and phone numbers of Mom's doctors, or keeping up with her ever-changing regimen of medications and doses, having the information readily available is important. And it all starts with knowing her date of birth, social security number, address, and phone number.

I know from the beginning I need to be organized and have a system. From discharge papers to elder care brochures, from passwords to PT exercises—I keep it all. Initially, everything seems important. I crave information, and anyone willing to share their knowledge, I gratefully accept. Eventually, I sort through what's worth keeping and what to toss, but one thing is for certain, I must document it all. So, I turn to Excel where I can organize data by tabs.

Two Journals: Keeping Up with Medical and Financial Information

What starts as a single Excel file capturing a medical chronology quickly becomes two files:

File 1: Medical Information

File 2: Financial Information

Just as important as it is to track medical info, what she's allergic to, when she had her last flu shot, and what her normal blood pressure readings are, it is equally important to know banking information, credit card details, automobile policy renewals, and how to access her online accounts.

While Mom is in the hospital, bills still need paying, grass needs mowing and homeowners' insurance needs renewing. Managing household responsibilities don't stop, and collecting information early on keeps things running smoothly. This is true whether she is living in her home or whether she's in a facility. Having account details allows me to conduct business on her behalf.

Mom has a living trust, and both my sister and I are powers of attorney, and as great as this sounds, navigating the maze of getting a customer service rep on the phone in today's world of automation is challenging. Then, when I do finally get a human on the line, explaining that I have power of attorney (POA) and can act on my mom's behalf is painful. Often, this exercise is more effort than I can muster, so I *magically* become Marlene. Sometimes impersonating her to get the cable bill paid is the easiest way to get things done. [This is not legal advice. Each situation is unique and may require consulting counsel for guidance.]

As much as I appreciate cyber security precautions in place protecting us from bad actors, these same barriers can stand in the way of helping to manage an aging parent's affairs when they are incapacitated. Having power of attorney and following the proper channels is the legitimate way to act on a parent's behalf, but desperate times can call for desperate measures.

For legal advice, consult an elder law attorney or advisor. They can offer guidance tailored to your family's situation and help you anticipate the bureaucratic hoops you'll inevitably have to jump through.

In the end, what I've learned through my journey is that strategy and creative problem-solving sometimes work best. Addressing the matter at hand, scratching something off the to-do list, and moving on is often the most efficient and satisfying approach.

Tracking Medical Details: Staying on Top of Allergies, Medications, and Physicians

Online apps accessible from a smart device might be the perfect solution. Since my sister and I share responsibility, having real-time access to a shared file works best for us, keeping us aligned and organized. Password protecting a file like this with sensitive, personal, proprietary information is a must. If unsure how to set this up, try searching "how to password protect an Excel file" using an AI assistant or search engine.

If leveraging technology isn't right for you, information can be tracked using a notebook or spiral binder. Whatever means you choose to use, make sure information is labeled, sectioned, legible, and easily accessible.

Here's a look at medical journal details and the information tracked.

Medical Information Tabs

Tab 1 - Patient Details

Tab 2–Current Medications

Tab 3–Allergies

Tab 4–Physicians

Tab 5–Facilities/Support Resources

Tab 6–Non-Allergic Meds

Tab 7–Chronology

PATIENT DETAILS

These are personal demographics like name, date of birth, height, weight, personal history, family history, and surgeries. Even though Mom denies her father's alcoholism or her own historical issues, it doesn't mean it wasn't real. I capture these details, so the medical staff has a clear, complete medical history of her physiological and psychological makeup.

CURRENT MEDICATIONS

This table tracks prescriptions and dosages, serving as both a living record and a quick reference for every medical professional we encounter—from hospital admissions to rehab intake—who inevitably ask, "What medications is she taking?"

The notes column is especially valuable. It captures important details like adverse reactions or sensitivities. Over time, as the years blur together, it becomes harder to recall exactly when she broke her hip or which medication triggered that intense bout of hives. Having it documented helps us stay accurate, responsive, and ready no matter who's asking.

Keeping a detailed timeline of prescribed medications is absolutely essential. She's extremely sensitive even to minor changes. Something as subtle as switching from a name-brand to a generic version can trigger a reaction. Her blood pressure meds are especially delicate: too strong, and she risks fainting and falling; too weak, and her numbers could spike, putting her at risk for a stroke.

Managing this "Goldilocks" mix—not too much, not too little, just right—has become one of the most critical roles in managing Mom's aging health journey. We face a constant balancing act, but a critical, necessary one.

ALLERGIES

Mom has a long list of allergies—everything from bee stings to beta blockers. In this tab, I include pictures showing what happens when she takes certain medications. It's taken time, trial, and more than a few scares to figure out what her body can and cannot tolerate.

In one instance, before we became intimately involved with her healthcare needs, she had a cardiologist who kept upping her dose of beta blockers. She ballooned up, swollen and unrecognizable, and we genuinely feared we were going to lose her.

How could we have let that happen? It was a case of "Not listening to the patient." Mom is a chronic complainer, and her low pain tolerance, at times, leads my sister, me, and even medical professionals to tune her out. We dismiss her discomfort as exaggeration. But in this case, it was nearly fatal. She turned out to be anaphylactic to beta blockers, and the continued dosage increases were, literally, poisoning her. Now, we listen differently and document everything.

> *Be aware of your blind spots. Sometimes we are too close to the patient, and we stop listening. If you are partnering in the care of a parent, someone needs to play the role of devil's advocate.*

In our case, if my sister discounts a complaint as 'Mom is being overly dramatic,' I take the opposing viewpoint. I ask, "Are you sure? I can see how she might feel that way." My sister does the same in reverse. When

I want to give up because I can't please Mom and I feel there is nothing more I can do, Tina challenges me to think differently and provides an alternative point of view.

Taking opposing positions for the patient's well-being is good, but it can create a strain on care team member relationships. Maintaining objectivity and minimizing emotions is difficult, and often it is exactly what is needed for the good of the patient.

Grant yourself grace. You will lose your temper. You will feel defeated. Step away. Get some air. Journal about the situation. Take the time you need to re-group.

Remember: the role of project manager of an aging loved one's life is a marathon, not a sprint.

PHYSICIANS

This next tab documents the medical team—names, specialties, contact info, and notes. Depending on the crisis of the month, the tab order shifts. When we're adjusting her blood pressure meds, the *Current Medications* tab takes priority. When we're searching for a new specialist, the Physicians tab moves to the front. The spreadsheet is a living document, constantly reshuffled to meet the needs of the moment.

Organize the tabs within the Excel workbook as needed. If you need an Excel refresher course, consider an online video or blog such as this Excel Essentials site, Basics of Excel (In Easy Steps) (excel-easy.com).

The *Physicians* tab includes key columns like Specialty, Name, Group/ Associates, Mailing Address, Phone, Email/Website, Hours, and Notes. I even copy and paste the physician's picture. But the real magic is in the details, capturing names of office managers, nurses, and support staff. Remember, the healthcare journey relies heavily on relationship-building. The more names I know, the smoother the interactions become.

Beyond physicians and specialists, I also log physical therapists, occupational therapists, speech therapists, and visiting nurses. These contacts are invaluable when rescheduling appointments or checking on progress. I can't emphasize this enough: relationships matter. Document names. Use them.

Getting past the gatekeeper is likely more successful when asking for a specific person in the office by name. And once connected with the right person, be warm, be respectful, and use their name. Kindness—a sometimes forgotten skill, opens doors, and makes all the difference.

If you aren't listed on the Health Insurance Portability and Accountability Act (HIPAA) release forms for hospitals, doctors or care facilities, get your name added. Without it, you won't have access to medical or financial information, and you may be blocked from receiving updates if a loved one is in the hospital or care setting.

Even with a medical power of attorney (MPOA) in place, a HIPAA release form is still required because the POA doesn't take effect until the patient is legally deemed unable to make their own medical decisions. In Mom's case, she's still capable of making decisions, with guidance from my sister and me, so we haven't activated the MPOA. This means medical and administrative staff can't legally share health or financial information with us unless our names are listed on the HIPAA form at each provider's office and at the hospital.

Thankfully, Mom understands the importance of this HIPAA form and makes sure both my sister and I are listed, but I always double-check. This is Project Management 101: plan for the unexpected and reduce risk. Without access to critical information, we can't make informed decisions or anticipate what's next. As Ronald Reagan said, "Trust, but verify."

If managing a parent's medical affairs solo, think ahead. Who else can step in if you're unavailable? Consider adding a son-in-law, daughter-in-law, trusted friend, or longtime neighbor to the HIPAA form. It's a simple step that can prevent major delays when time and clarity matter most.

Non-Allergic Meds

As mentioned, Mom is highly sensitive to medications, so when there's a need for a new, short-term antibiotic, we are hyper vigilant. A low dose with a Benadryl chaser is our normal process to avoid a hives breakout or ulcers forming. When we discover a med that works and she doesn't have an adverse reaction, I document it. Her next upper respiratory infection may call for an antibiotic, and having these details is helpful.

Once Mom had such a visceral reaction to a medication that it took four months with weekly appointments to a skin specialist treating and re-wrapping her legs with compression bandages to heal her skin. Micro-managing her meds makes life more manageable for us and mitigates the risk of new ailments for Mom.

This non-allergic meds tab may be less beneficial to you, but there may be an equally important topic that needs tracking. Think about the medical details you need to keep up with and add a tab. This is a working document to help you as project manager of your loved one's life.

Facilities / Support Resources

This tab tracks care resources such as rehab centers, respite care facilities, home health services, and more. Column headings include: Company, Service, and Phone.

Whenever I visit a facility, even if we don't end up using it, I document what I learn. This project manager role is for the long haul, and there's no way I'll remember every place I've toured or every person I've spoken with. I may run across a service that Mom may not need today, but she might need in the future, so I keep track of it. If a facility stands out, for better or worse, I document these notes, too.

Any time I receive a business card, brochure, or email with direct contact info, especially mobile numbers, I log it. These connections often become lifelines in a future phase of this aging-parent marathon.

One more thing to keep in mind, the elder care community is surprisingly small. Staff rotate between facilities, and they talk. Be sure not to burn bridges along the way. Relationships matter. Names open doors.

Along with tracking details in the shared Excel file, I also save names, titles, and facility affiliations directly into my phone contacts. It's a small habit with big payoffs. Early in my role as project manager of Mom's life, I met a business manager at an assisted living facility. I logged her name along with the facility name, then moved on.

Keep notes and names. You never know when you might need to refer to them. Associate facility names with contacts you meet. Complete as many of the fields on the contact page on your phone as possible, including facility addresses, websites, contact name and title. In the future, when you search for someone, you may not remember their name, but you might remember the facility name or the street where it is located.

Also, don't be shy about texting or calling people you meet along the way. People want to help. They don't mind passing your name along or sharing a resource or a list of facilities. If you don't get a response to an email or text, take a different approach.

Years later, we found ourselves in a familiar rinse-and-repeat cycle. Mom needed another recovery stay after a hospital discharge. Thanks to saving the business manager's name along with the facility name in my phone contacts, I found her easily. I sent a quick text to reintroduce myself and ask if she was still at the facility.

Her reply? "No, I've moved out of state, but I still keep in touch with folks there. It was a great place to work and a quality place for elders. Let me send you a contact number. Can I pass along your name and number?"

Just like that, I was back in business. Relationships matter, and a well-organized contact list can be a powerful tool. Build rapport, make connections, and pay it forward. Share information and resources gathered along the way. Formal and informal social networks in the elder care space are invaluable.

Chronology Journal

This tab functions as a journal, a place to track patterns, reactions, and clues that help uncover the root cause of Mom's medical issues. When ulcers appear on her legs or her face turns fire red and swollen, I log the medications she's taking, note the timing of her last dose, and document it with photos.

Mom despises having her picture taken even when she's dressed up and feeling good. Capturing her image when she's sick earns me a sharp glare and a muttered string of curses. Still, these photos matter. They tell a story that words alone can't convey. For current and future physicians, visual documentation offers a visceral understanding of how her body responds to medications she can't tolerate. It's not just record keeping—it's evidence.

Along with pictures associated with allergic reactions, I also track blood pressure readings. Her blood pressure swings erratically from high to low, back to high again. Documenting blood pressure readings, along with the times of day that she's taking her medication, paints another important picture for the doctors. *Does she need greater or fewer milligrams of a medication? Do we need to spread out the frequency with which she's taking it? Does it matter if she's taking the medicine after eating a meal?* Capturing these patterns equips doctors with the insight they need to make informed decisions and help us help her.

Journal what's important. You may choose to journal episodes of memory lapse, glucose numbers, or weight changes. Data is valuable, and knowledge is power. You can't manage what you don't know. You don't have to keep the journal forever. That can be overwhelming and unrealistic, but if you are trying to track down a behavior issue or deduce a medical anomaly, capturing chronological events can help.

Managing Financial Information: A Key Role in Coordinated Care

Just as a medical journal is essential, so too is a financial journal. Excel is a reliable tool for organizing this kind of data—its tab structure and formula functions make it ideal for tracking income and expenses.

Because this journal contains confidential and sensitive information, it's critical to password-protect the file. It includes personally identifiable information (PII), which refers to data that can uniquely identify an individual on its own or when combined with other details. PII is highly sensitive and must be handled with care. Examples include:

Full name

Social Security number (SSN)

Driver's license number

Mailing address

Credit card information

Protecting this data isn't just good practice; it's a critical security safeguard. If encryption and/or password protecting a file is unfamiliar, research the process before documenting financial data. For a tutorial on protecting an Excel file, see: *Project an Excel file - Microsoft Support.*

A finance journal might include the following tabs:

Tab 1—Investments & Banking

Tab 2–Account Logins

Tab 3–Recurring Expenses

Tab 4–Attorney Info

INVESTMENTS & BANKING

The investments and banking tab tracks active financial accounts and overall stability. Managing monthly expenses, from lawn care to utility bills, is part of the day-to-day management of Mom's household. Alongside these immediate needs, it's also important to monitor the investment accounts she and Dad built over their working years. Her Social Security income, combined with investment distributions, forms the foundation of her financial solvency.

Each month, funds from her retirement accounts are deposited as Required Minimum Distributions (RMDs), the mandated withdrawal from certain retirement plans once a person reaches a specific age. Before her health started declining, Mom withdrew the full RMD in December and relied on Social Security for the rest of the year. But as care needs have grown, whether in-home support or facility-based expenses, a single annual withdrawal no longer suffices.

To keep pace with rising medical costs, we've shifted to monthly withdrawals, spreading her RMDs throughout the year. To avoid a hefty tax bill in April, the financial institution withholds a portion of each withdrawal, reducing the net amount deposited into her checking account. Managing Mom's income effectively is a balancing act of ensuring steady cash flow while staying ahead of tax obligations.

This resource is not intended to provide financial guidance. To understand how best to handle income and expenses for your situation, consult a financial advisor.

Consulting a financial advisor is key to finding the right strategy. In our case, maintaining a steady stream of income to offset ongoing expenses has proven most effective.

In addition to columns like Phone, Account, Contact, Login, Address, and Website, I regularly log account balances, too, including checking, savings, and investments.

Tracking these figures over time reveals trends and market shifts that guide decision-making. It's hard to manage what isn't visible, and having a clear picture of financial standing brings a sense of order. Just like with medical data, financial insight is empowering.

Understanding her financial position helps shape decisions about care. This is part of a constant balancing act, ensuring she receives the social and emotional support she needs, while preserving her resources and honoring her wishes, all while being good stewards of her hard-earned money.

ACCOUNT LOGINS

Along with managing bank accounts and investments, keeping up with all the account logins and passwords brings a sense of order and control. Whether handling everything solo or coordinating with siblings, full visibility into her affairs is essential. Not only does it provide a check and balance, but it also establishes shared roles and responsibilities. Having online access to accounts also allows access to pay Mom's bills and monitor unauthorized charges.

My sister and I brainstorm the variety of accounts she has and log the information. For example, accounts to consider include:

Life insurance policy information

Credit cards

Medicare card (include front and back image of the card)

Supplemental insurance (include front and back images of the card)

Prescription drug coverage (if different from Medicare coverage)

Electronic Health Record (EHR) portals like MyChart or FollowMyHealth

Apple or Google account

Amazon account

Managing matters online provides a layer of anonymity. There are no phone screeners or voice recognition barriers. You can get in, take care of business, and move on. When you are helping manage an aging parent's affairs, navigating security hurdles can feel daunting, and using online access can be easier and more efficient.

Keep in mind that many online accounts require multi-factor authentication. When prompted, a code is sent to an email address or texted to a phone and must be entered as a second layer of security in addition to the password. If you are partnering with a sibling, make sure both of your contact options are listed. For example, if my sister needs a code to log in, her phone number must be included along with mine.

RECURRING EXPENSES

This tab is dedicated to tracking ongoing financial commitments, distinct from general banking and one-time expenses. It provides a clear view of predictable outflows, which is helpful for budgeting and long-term planning. Column headings include: Company, Service, Phone, Account Number, Address, Contact, Expense and Frequency.

Capturing details in one centralized place makes it easier to spot patterns, flag changes, and avoid costly oversights, especially when coordinating care across multiple providers. Attention to detail and thorough documentation are essential skills for any project manager. Whether it's the name of the HOA president or the timing of her next pest control visit, even the most obscure details can become unexpectedly important.

ATTORNEY INFO

This tab contains attorney information. Our initial contact with an elder law attorney occurred shortly after Dad died when Mom needed to update her living trust. Since it may be weeks, months or years between events when needing to contact the elder law attorney, having the information readily available when needed is critical. Similar to other tabs, column headings on this tab include: Name/Firm, Address, Phone, Website, Notes.

LIVING TRUST

The last tab of the finance journal is information about my parents' living trust. Along with the hard copy binder of the living trust, some important segments are copied into this financial journal for quick, easy access.

**This content is not intended as legal advice.
Each situation is unique, and the appropriate legal path
should be determined based on individual circumstances.**

Demystifying the Living Trust: What It Is and Why It Matters

Living trusts can get complicated and knowing what's important versus what is boilerplate information that can be skimmed over can be confusing. What I determine is that there are three key sections pertinent to our needs: Medical Power of Attorney (MPOA); Financial Power of Attorney (FPOA); and Certification of Intent.

Activating a Medical Power of Attorney (MPOA) signifies that the individual is no longer able to make medical decisions independently. For us, this feels like a last-resort measure. Since Mom remains lucid and capable of speaking for herself, we've chosen not to invoke the MPOA. As a result, the attending physician at the nursing home refuses to engage with me or my sister, despite our deep involvement in her care.

> A medical power of attorney (MPOA) (sometimes called a healthcare proxy or healthcare agent designation) is a legal document that allows someone you trust to make medical decisions if you cannot. It applies broadly to all healthcare settings—hospitals, nursing homes, clinics, or even at home with hospice care. The authority is not limited to one facility type; it follows the person wherever they receive care.
>
> Leveraging a MPOA in a hospital setting empowers your agent to make decisions about surgeries, treatments, medications, or life-support measures. Whereas in a nursing home, the MPOA may focus more on long-term care, daily living needs, and end-of-life choices.

This tension reflects a broader challenge: balancing Mom's autonomy with the need for informed advocacy. We want her to retain control over her medical choices for as long as possible, yet our historical insight into her health and behavior can help guide clinical decisions. Even though we're listed on the HIPAA release form, the physician communicates solely with her and the facility staff, leaving us out of the loop.

Another challenging, necessary, and often misunderstood element of leveraging a living trust is the financial power of attorney (FPOA). This is also commonly referred to as the financial durable power of attorney (FDPOA). Even with a copy of the documents in hand, when visiting the local cable provider to pick up new equipment on Mom's behalf, I was met with resistance. I provided the financial POA information, and neither the associate nor the manager knew what to do with it. As critical and invaluable as it is to have a POA, those requesting it might not know what to do with it.

> *Ask questions and research all you can about a living trust or whatever means you have for handling an elder's affairs. Ask your legal advisor questions such as:*
>
> • *Do we need to list the bank account and all investment accounts in the trust? Why or why not?*
>
> • *Are there additional actions we need to address with Mom's accounts? What's the relationship between the beneficiaries of accounts and trustees?*
>
> • *If there are two people listed as co-trustees, does it make matters harder? Why or why not?*

PAYABLE ON DEATH AND TRANSFER ON DEATH

Interesting fact. Who knew that Power of Attorney (POA) is void at the point of death? I had no idea. When a person passes, the phrases Transfer On Death (TOD) and Payable On Death (POD) supersede POA.

Transfer on Death (TOD):

This designation allows an account holder to pass assets from brokerage accounts, stocks, and bonds directly to beneficiaries upon their death, bypassing probate. TOD applies to securities and security-related assets.

Payable on Death (POD)

A payable on death (POD) account is a legal arrangement that allows an account owner to designate a beneficiary. This can occur at the point at which the account is set up or afterwards. The purpose of a POD account is to keep the money out of probate court, simplifying the transfer process.

Converting an account to a POD account is straightforward. The account holder notifies their bank of the chosen beneficiary, and the bank provides a beneficiary designation form.

While the account holder is alive, the named beneficiary has no access to the funds.

The role of project manager of Mom's life requires keen organization, strategic thinking, skilled negotiation—and above all, tremendous compassion. I navigate it all while tending to my own family's needs and leading initiatives in my professional life. Managing Mom's care isn't a side gig. It's a full-scale, unpaid project with real stakes and constant demands. And while the title may be unofficial, the responsibility is anything but.

CHAPTER 4

Get Ready, Rehab is Next

Topics

— **From Hospital to Healing: Preparing
for What Comes Next**

— **Not Always the Answer: When a Social Worker
Falls Short**

— **Rehab Choices Matter: Understanding Your Options**

Caring for an aging parent is often an unpredictable journey. Whether it unfolds suddenly, like mine with my mom falling and being rushed to the hospital, or whether it develops gradually over time, figuring out 'what comes next' when coordinating care is often a mystery.

This was certainly true with my mom's first hospital stay. She arrived at the emergency room by ambulance, dehydrated, semi-conscious and in urgent need of care. The medical team immediately focused on stabilizing her: replenishing fluids, controlling her blood pressure, and checking for signs of organ damage. She was admitted, and after several days of intensive treatment, ensuring she was out of danger, a critical issue surfaced—Mom had a broken hip that would require surgical repair and a long recovery.

Luckily, she makes it through hip replacement surgery complication-free, but then, I am blindsided by a new challenge that I hadn't even considered: *Where will Mom go when she's discharged?* The reality of post-hospital care hits me head-on. I am faced with exploring rehabilitation options, determining available resources and figuring out essential questions to ask.

From Hospital to Healing: Preparing for What Comes Next

SURGERY DAY

Mom is restless and weary. She's been in the hospital for three weeks. Constant monitoring, endless prodding, and the inability to get a good night's rest can wear anyone down, but for Mom, who is easily irritated, it's especially draining.

Today is surgery day to fix her broken hip. Dr. Riley stops by, confirming her pre-op bloodwork looks good and everything is set. Something is added to her IV to help her relax, and soon she's dozing off. Tina and I lean in, kiss her, and whisper, 'We love you,' and reassure her we will see her soon. The nurse releases the brakes on the bed and wheels her out of the room.

We settle into the waiting room, and Tina's phone vibrates.

"They need to see us in pre-op," she says. *They've not had time to even start the surgery. What could they need from us? Did she have a stroke or a heart attack?* We push through the double doors and head to Mom's pre-op bay.

The nurse reassures us, "Your mom is fine. We just discovered she has a slight arrhythmia."

Arrhythmia is a term used to describe any irregularity in the rate or rhythm of a person's heartbeat. It occurs when the heart's electrical impulses become too fast, too slow, or erratic, leading to an abnormal heartbeat. When the heart can't beat properly, it doesn't pump blood efficiently. As a result, vital organs like the lungs, brain, and others may struggle to function, potentially leading to damage or shutdown.

"So, can she still have surgery?" I ask.

"It is a risk, but given that it is a slight arrhythmia and she could have been living with this her entire life without an issue, we should be fine moving forward with the surgery. We just want you to be aware of the situation, and we need consent to continue."

We all agree to move forward with the surgery, as the risk seems minimal, and Mom wants to get back on her feet to resume her normal, active life.

Surgery goes well, and afterwards, Mom returns to her room.

PREPARING FOR DISCHARGE

The next morning, as usual, I'm up early and at Mom's bedside. Shortly after eight, the first hospital staff person, the social worker, enters the room. She introduces herself, and we exchange niceties. Facing Mom, she says, "Your surgery went well, and we have discharge orders for the next day or so. You are going home."

"What?" I blurt out, my unfiltered response more aggressive than I intend. I continue. "No. She can't go home. She can't even walk. She can't get to the toilet. She's seventy-eight years old, and she lives alone. She just had surgery. No. She's not going home," I insist.

Ignoring me, the social worker gently lifts Mom's hand and squeezes it. As her body language screams *insensitive, uncaring daughter,* she says, "Well, if she can't go home with you, then the only option is a rehab facility."

I attempt to regain my composure. "I'm sorry for my outburst," I say. "It's been a long couple of weeks. You see, I don't live here. I'm from Texas. And my sister can't stay with her, either."

More disapproving looks. My effort to smooth things over isn't landing. It is obvious she believes Mom should recover at home, and that someone should move in with her until she's back on her feet. Sensing that scenario is not going to happen, she acquiesces. "Well, then you'll need a place for her to be discharged to, likely by Thursday."

Thursday? That's two days from now.

"How do we find a place?" I ask.

She pulls a pamphlet from her pocket and thrusts it in my direction.

"There is a list of places on the last two pages," she says. "Some might be out of business or not accepting patients. You'll need to call them and find out."

She is of little help, but I've got my assignment, and a deadline. I need to find a place—now. I need to do some research, and I need to do it fast.

I can't stress this enough! Be nice. Making enemies with people who can help may make things harder than they need to be. Pause. Take a deep breath. And keep emotions intact. It will pay off in the long run.

Not Always the Answer: When a Social Worker Falls Short

ROLE OF A HOSPITAL SOCIAL WORKER

As a point of reference, hospital social workers typically help patients and their families obtain resources and offer support as patients recover from injury or illness. They often coordinate with rehab facilities and determine space availability.

Responsibilities may include:

Comprehensive Assessment—Conducts psychosocial evaluations to understand a patient's social, emotional, and financial needs, often through interviews with patients, families and medical professionals.

Individualized Case Management—Develops and implements personalized care plans, coordinating with medical teams to ensure well-rounded patient support.

Resource Navigation—Assists patients in accessing healthcare services, financial aid, transportation, and medication support.

Discharge Planning—Coordinates post-hospital care, scheduling follow-up appointments, arranging home health services, and ensuring a smooth transition.

Patient Advocacy—Protects patients' rights, helping them make informed decisions and ensuring their voices are heard within the healthcare system.

Education and Awareness—Informs patients and families about medical conditions, treatment options, and resources.

Collaborative Care—Works alongside physicians, nurses, and case managers to provide coordinated, holistic patient care.

Many people assume that once a social worker is involved, they will take full ownership of the transition, making calls, arranging placements, and guiding the entire process. It is often a hands-off experience for many families. This isn't the case for us.

Throughout Mom's recovery journey, we work with various social workers—both in hospitals and senior living communities. While some are more effective than others, none fully meet our expectations. To be fair, we have high standards. Simply finding the next available open bed isn't enough. We want to be sure it aligns with our criteria for safety, quality, and compatibility with Mom's medical needs and personality. So, we take on a more active role, often stepping into responsibilities typically handled by a patient care coordinator or social worker.

On a Mission—Find Mom a Rehab Facility

With the pamphlet in hand, I begin researching rehab facilities online. My priority is checking online reviews, and I eliminate any with an average of two or three stars.

I also focus on facilities that are close to Mom's and my sister's houses. Mom needs to be close by so we can drop in during the day in between conference calls and work demands. After narrowing the search, three rehab facilities remain, all within skilled nursing centers. These locations focus on short-term rehabilitation rather than long-term residency, offering patients the opportunity to recover before returning home or transitioning to senior living communities.

The staff at a rehab facility may include registered nurses, licensed practical and vocational nurses, physical and speech therapists, audiologists, a medical director, and other specialized healthcare professionals. And, since rehab centers operate under strict state and federal regulations, they must meet local compliance standards as Medicare Part A coverage typically allows up to 100 days within a rehab facility as deemed necessary.

Take time to explore the different parts of Medicare, as each covers distinct aspects of healthcare:

Part A handles hospital stays and facility fees—think of it like room and board.

Part B covers outpatient care, such as doctor visits, physical therapy, and occupational therapy.

Part C, known as Medicare Advantage, is bundled Medicare Part A and B, an alternative offered by private insurers that may include additional benefits such as dental, vision and/or prescription drug coverage.

Part D covers prescription drugs.

Be mindful of deductibles, co-pays, and limitations on length of stay. Coverage varies. Some individuals have standard Medicare (Parts A and B), while others opt for Advantage Plans (Part C) or add prescription coverage (Part D). Be sure to review the elder's specific plan, including any supplemental coverage.

In our mom's situation–recovering in a rehab facility–we can anticipate Medicare Part A charges for the 'room and board,' Medicare Part B charges for therapy services she receives, and Medicare Part D charges for prescriptions.

A single, easy-to-use resource for exploring health care options is available on the Medicare.gov website. Instead of navigating multiple sites, the Centers for Medicare and Medicaid Services (CMS) offers a Care Compare tool, where you can explore information about doctors, hospitals and inpatient rehab facilities. The tool provides data on cost, quality of care, service volume, and more, helping patients and caregivers make well-informed decisions. Users can even select several facilities at once to compare their performance across key quality measures. Find Healthcare Providers: Compare Care Near You | Medicare.

SCHEDULING REHAB FACILITY VISITS

Now that I have a list of three facilities, it's time to schedule visits. I call each location, ask about availability, request a site visit and tour, and brief them on Mom's situation. Often, the conversation evolves into her backstory—how she lay on the floor for four days, spent weeks in the hospital, and recently underwent hip replacement surgery. Providing context is essential. While the primary focus is rehabilitating her hip, occupational therapy and a cognitive assessment may also be necessary. She's doing well overall, but at times, I notice her slipping into illogical dialogue and dementia-like episodes that require monitoring.

My first question is always, "Do you have availability?" Mom is set to leave the hospital in a few days, and if they aren't accepting new patients, there's no point in scheduling a visit. The response is often the same: "We don't have availability today, but one of our rehab patients may be leaving tomorrow. Things change daily, sometimes hourly, here."

This answer frustrates me. I thrive on structure, planning and order, and phrases like "we might have space" amp up my anxiety. This is an ongoing battle throughout Mom's care journey. One I grow accustomed to, but never fully accept.

Rehab Choices Matter: Understanding Your Options

Despite facilities passing an initial online review, each presents vastly different realities. Site visits are essential.

One facility feels old, dark, and dreary, seemingly untouched for years. Drab curtains, dim lighting, and nicked paneling bring to mind the basement of my childhood home–last remodeled in the mid-seventies. And it's not a stylish mid-century-modern (MCM) revival; no, it's original MCM fare.

Another facility has stellar ratings, glowing reviews, and praise for its staff. I'm hopeful, but during my visit, something still feels off. It resembles a converted hospital, with semi-private rooms and elderly patients asleep in wheelchairs along the hallway corridors. A visit to the 'gym' where Mom will have physical therapy is cramped and difficult to navigate.

Discouraged, I step into the lobby of the last location on my list. Immediately, I'm struck by how different this place looks. Picture a fifties diner, popcorn Thursdays, and bingo every afternoon at three. This place is as good as a transatlantic cruise, except it's a nursing home. Instead of Cruise Director Julie McCoy, there's "Social Worker Joyce," orchestrating the 'Move-Them-In, Move-Them-Out' process. Purser Jeremy handles bedpan duty.

This facility has a different vibe than the others. Just off the lobby, a gas-burning fireplace flickers, and the festive scent of pine fills the air. A beautifully decorated Christmas tree stands just inside the dining area. During the tour, I notice the wide hallways. Residents aren't sitting slumped in their wheelchairs but rather scooting along with purpose, gathering in the activity room for a Christmas carol sing-along.

My tour guide, Social Worker Joyce, shows me an available semi-private room. She points out that a solid wall separates the two residents, though they share a bathroom. In my excitement over all the 'pluses,' it doesn't register for me that Mom's suite mate's TV is blaring, full volume—a missed detail I grow to regret.

Consider whether a private or semi-private room is best. Sharing a room ultimately was not a good solution for Mom.

My tour wraps up with a stop at the spacious gym, equipped with everything from mats and Bosu balls to hand weights, massage tables, and step platforms, rivaling a private physical therapy studio. The impressive setup highlights the true purpose of rehab: helping Mom regain strength, build muscle, and ultimately walk with confidence again.

"I'm sold. Where do I sign?" I ask.

"No need to sign anything," Joyce says. "You've already given me your mom's name and date of birth. Just let the hospital social worker know your mom will be coming here for rehab, and we'll take care of the rest."

Nirvana. Someone who is actually helpful coordinating Mom's care.

I snap a few pictures of the dining room, lobby, the nurses' station, and Mom's semi-private room. Since she struggles to see images on my phone, I print them so she can get a sense of where she's headed after she's discharged, hopeful of easing her anxiety and making the transition smoother.

Before pulling out of the parking lot, I close my eyes and lean my head back. Mission accomplished. In less than twenty-four hours, Mom has a spot in a rehab facility that feels safe, clean, and perfectly equipped for her recovery.

Questions to Ask When Visiting Rehab Facilities

FACILITY AND CARE SERVICES

What type of rehabilitation services does the facility provide?

How often are physical therapy, occupational therapy, and other services offered?

What is the staff-to-patient ratio, and how experienced are the caregivers?

DAILY LIFE AND ACCOMMODATIONS

What amenities are available, such as private rooms, dining options, or recreational activities?

Can family members visit and are there restrictions on visiting hours?

What personal items should we bring?

INSURANCE AND FINANCIAL CONSIDERATIONS

What costs should we expect, and what is covered by insurance?

Are financial assistance programs available?

What happens if the stay extends longer than originally planned?

TRANSITION AND DISCHARGE PLANNING

How is patient progress measured, and who determines when it is time to leave?

Is there a typical length of time that rehab lasts? Is it days, weeks or months?

What support is needed when transitioning back home?

ALTERNATIVE TO REHABILITATING IN A FACILITY—IN-HOME CARE

A rehab alternative we did not opt for was discharging Mom from the hospital directly to her home. Since I live out of state and Tina juggles full-time work and family responsibilities, in-home rehab simply wasn't an option for us. We could have opted to pay full-time caregivers, but that requires really deep pockets, which wasn't feasible for us as is the case for others.

In-home rehab requires greater coordination among family members and service providers and often demands a more hands-on approach. Typically, an in-home evaluation is arranged, during which a registered nurse assesses the home and recommends modifications for safety. Depending on physician orders and coordination with a home care service provider, patients can receive physical therapy, occupational therapy, speech therapy, and nursing support which are usually covered under Medicare Part B.

Questions to Ask the Hospital Social Worker if Rehabilitating at Home

What kind of assistance will be needed at home?

Is home health care or physical therapy available, and how is it arranged?

Is personal care available to assist with bathing/showering, dressing, toileting, companionship, and how is it arranged?

How is medical equipment, such as a walker or grab bars, obtained?

What if pain or complications occur after discharge?

Safety and Mobility

How can the home be made safer to prevent falls?

Are there transportation services available for follow-up appointments?

Medication and Pain Management

What pain medications are being prescribed, and are there side effects to watch for?

Will prescriptions be sent to the pharmacy, or do they need to be picked up?

Can prescriptions be delivered?

Financial and Insurance Considerations

Does insurance cover home health services or rehabilitation?

Are there financial assistance programs available?

INPATIENT REHAB FACILITIES (IRFs)—ANOTHER OPTION

An alternative to skilled nursing centers with rehab facilities is a dedicated Inpatient Rehab Facility (IRF). IRFs provide intensive therapy and medical supervision for patients recovering from major health events, helping them rebuild strength and regain independence.

Unlike skilled nursing facilities (SNFs), which focus on long-term recovery or maintenance care, IRFs emphasize short-term rehabilitation through structured, high-intensity therapy programs tailored to individual recovery goals. A key distinction between an IRF and an SNF is the intensity of therapy. Patients in an IRF must be able to participate in at least three hours of therapy per day, five to seven days a week.

This structured approach includes physical therapy, occupational therapy, and, when needed, speech therapy, all designed to speed up recovery. A helpful resource for comparing an SNF and an IRF for rehab can be found on the exacare.com website in the inpatient-rehab-skilled-nursing-facility article.

SENIOR-CENTRIC INPATIENT REHAB FACILITY

A third inpatient rehab facility option is a senior-focused short-term rehab facility. This is a newer model and an alternative to a SNF rehab center with less intensity than an IRF rehab facility. Research shows that patients in facilities with an institutionalized atmosphere struggle to regain full strength effectively. One way this newer short-term senior rehab model sets itself apart is by offering specialized care, state-of-the-art amenities, and a personalized, supportive environment tailored to each patient's needs.

Staff members are trained in geriatric care, prepared to assist aging adults recovering from knee and joint replacements, complex IV therapies, advanced wound care, dialysis, cardiopulmonary issues, and more. By integrating skilled nursing services, these facilities allow patients to transition from hospital care more quickly while still receiving quality medical support. Many also provide private rooms with private bathrooms.

> Over the course of Mom's journey, I had the luxury of leveraging learned skills more than once. It was like Groundhog Day with a medical twist: *the bad news was that it happened again, but the good news was that we knew what to do.* When Mom experienced a second hip fracture, (she broke her other hip just four months after returning home from the first ordeal) she was admitted to a traditional IRF with patients of varying ages. One was recovering from a debilitating motorcycle accident, and another was a young mother recovering from a stroke following childbirth.
>
> The therapy was demanding, but Mom loved it. With stamina and determination, she powered through four-hour-a-day sessions that might have overwhelmed others but proved to be just right for her. She moved through rehab with strength and resolve, earning praise along the way and ultimately returning home healthier and stronger.

LEVERAGING EXPERIENCE

With each of Mom's rehab experiences, I learn more and ask deeper, more thought-provoking questions. Depending on Mom's endurance, age, and injury, one facility may be a better fit than another. I also adjust my expectations of what a rehab center should offer. For instance, afternoon bingo and popcorn socials, while great for respite care, aren't as essential in a rehab setting.

Instead, our focus when selecting a rehab facility is on cleanliness, safety, staff training, and access to on-site PT, OT, and speech therapy. As we learn over time, rehab stays are short-term and we are less concerned about 'moving mom into a college dorm with a door wreath' and more about ensuring she is comfortable *enough* in her new surroundings where the priority is recovery and regaining mobility.

CHAPTER 5

Next Stop—Rehab

Topics

— Checking into Rehab: The Wheelchair Surprise

— Rehab Essentials: What to Pack
and What to Leave at Home

— Making Rehab Feel Like Home:
A Surefire Way to Get Staff to Stop In

— Communicating with the Staff:
How to Advocate Effectively for the Patient

— PT and OT Demystified:
How Therapy Helps Patients Get Back on Their Feet

— Wrapping Up Rehab Check-In

Mom is scheduled for discharge and heading to rehab. Despite having only two days to find and secure a facility, we pull it off, and I feel confident about where she's going. We've found a great facility with a large gym for PT and OT.

LEAVING THE HOSPITAL

Every day I spend navigating this role through Mom's care journey feels like a roller coaster ride—with highs, lows, and unexpected turns. A few days ago, I was nervous about her hip replacement surgery, then relieved it was a success and then panicked trying to find a place where she could rehab.

Today, the anxiety shifts. It's no longer the fear of Mom having a place to go that has my stomach churning, but the anticipation of what happens next. *Will Mom like the rehab center? Will she give the nurses a hard time?* She hates change and introducing her to unfamiliar staff and new surroundings is filled with uncertainty.

I've done everything I can to make this a smooth transition, including coordinating with the hospital's social worker, sharing pictures so Mom knows what to expect, and hyping the place up to build excitement. The next part is up to Mom. Her chariot, her minivan, awaits.

I've been away from home for three weeks. I missed Thanksgiving and pressed pause on my life with my husband and kids. But I see an escape route ahead. After we get Mom settled, I can fly home just in time for the pre-Christmas rush of shopping, wrapping, baking, and memory-making.

Not so fast.

Before we leave the hospital, a circus of chaos unfolds in Mom's room. Nurses, therapists, discharge coordinators. Everyone piles in, barking instructions: *Sign here. Take this. Don't forget that.* PT exercises, prescriptions, paperwork—it's all happening at once.

And just when I think we've got things under control, a young tech says: "You must be excited about going home."

I chime in quickly. "She's being discharged but not heading home. She's going to rehab."

Mom jumps in too, only she's combative, argumentative. She's still in her hospital gown, and we are already fighting about the rehab place. Thankfully, the chaos in the room works in our favor. Staff move around her to gather her belongings and help her dress. It's enough of a distraction to push through the moment. She is not happy, but she tolerates the commotion long enough for us to load her into the van.

Once we're on the road, I remind her of the pictures I showed her, the friendly staff I met, the impressive gym where she'll do her physical therapy. Little by little, the tension eases.

"I do love exercising," she admits. "If I can just get up and moving, I'll get better."

She's on board.

"Yes," I encourage her. "You just need some support, and the therapists will help you build up your strength."

For the first time today, she seems hopeful. Now, the challenge is holding onto that optimism.

Checking into Rehab: The Wheelchair Surprise

We pull up to the rehab center, and I tell Mom to stay in the car while I get her checked in. I buzz in, and as the secured door clicks open. I step into the lobby.

It's quiet. Nurses and staff are scarce. No one is in the front office to greet me. A few residents shuffle around, moving their wheelchairs with slow, deliberate motions, Fred Flintstone style. An elderly gentleman in a worn Cardinals sweatshirt smiles and waves sluggishly in my direction.

I later learn this is Leo, the resident greeter. Leo has the inside scoop on everyone: who's late for their shift, who stepped out for a smoke break, who's fighting with whom. Over time, I discover every facility has someone like Leo.

If you want to know what's really going on, get to know the resident watchdog. They'll fill you in on the staff, the families, even how mom is adjusting, whether she's getting along or causing trouble.

Along with Leo the greeter and the meandering residents, I notice something I hadn't before—everything is slower here. Life moves at a slower pace, like stepping back in time before self-driving cars, before everyone was glued to their cell phones, and before people relied on social media to figure out how to host a baby shower or assemble a snack platter.

Here, people make eye contact. They crave conversation and human touch. No one is in a hurry.

Eventually, I grow to appreciate the slower pace, bask in the love of simple rhythms, but right now, I'm on a mission. My frustration builds as

I wait impatiently for someone to help me.

Then, from around the corner, in walks someone I assume is the front office receptionist.

"Can I help you?" she asks.

I explain Mom is checking into room 101B. I tell her she is waiting outside.

"Okay. Bring her in," she says.

"I don't have a wheelchair, and I can't get her out of the van."

She pauses. "You don't have a wheelchair? Can she walk?"

"Umm, no," I bite my lip, holding back the sarcasm, and as much as I try to disguise my emotion, my response drips with contempt. "She just had hip surgery. She just left the hospital. She can't walk."

It's December. It's cold. I've been inside for ten minutes, and my mother, fresh out of a month-long hospital stay, sits alone in a van out front. I am dangerously close to snapping.

"Well, most residents bring their own wheelchairs or walkers. Sometimes we have a spare. Let me see if I can find one." She disappears again.

I exhale sharply, closing my eyes against the mounting irritation. Slowly, I open them again. Across the lobby, Leo waves and offers me a reassuring smile—a much-needed dose of compassion. I giggle, glance down at the floor, and shake my head.

Is this a warning sign? Should I find Mom somewhere else? No, I learn that this chaos is normal, and so is the unpredictability of whether care partners and elder care staff have critical thinking, problem-solving and proactive thinking skills.

After a brief wait, the social worker, Joyce, steps into the lobby, pushing a wheelchair. Apparently, she knows where the secret stash of equipment is stored.

"Nice to see you again. Where's Mom?" she says.

Finally, we are getting somewhere.

When coordinating rehab facility plans, ask if you are expected to provide any special equipment, such as a wheelchair or walker. If you don't own it, is this something the social worker at the hospital orders, or is it something the rehab facility arranges?

Rehab Essentials: What to Pack and What to Leave at Home

While in rehab, patients get up and dress for therapy daily. Be prepared with comfortable, loose-fitting clothing and personal essentials to ensure a smooth stay.

Packing List: Must Have Items for Rehab

Clothing and Footwear

- T-shirts
- Sweatpants or stretch pants
- Shorts (recommended for knee or leg surgery patients)
- Underwear, incontinence pads/underpants
- Socks
- Pajamas, a robe, and slippers with tread or traction
- Soft-soled or athletic shoes with nonskid soles (avoid sandals)

Toiletries and Personal Care

- Personal hygiene items
- Hairbrush or comb
- Shampoo and other hair care products
- Makeup or shaving kit
- Denture adhesive and cleaner, toothbrush and toothpaste
- Dentures, hearing aids, and/or glasses

Any assistive devices already owned,
such as a cane or walker

Primary care physician's name and contact information

A list of current medications (Do not bring medications
from home. Prescriptions are filled on-site with an
approved pharmacy.)

Prescription plan identification cards

A living will or advance directives, if applicable

Additional Items for Comfort and Convenience

Books, magazines, cards, or other activities for downtime

A small amount of cash (five dollars or less)

A notepad and pen for jotting down notes or valuable
information

Phone numbers of relatives, friends,
and emergency contacts

What NOT to bring

Perfumes, colognes, or scented lotions, due to allergies of
other patients and staff

Valuables such as expensive jewelry or family heirlooms

Substantial amounts of cash

Debit and credit cards

Medications

Making Rehab Feel Like Home: A Surefire Way to Get Staff to Stop In

SETTLING INTO HER ROOM

Knowing Mom will struggle adjusting to her new surroundings, I bring a few things from home, her beloved houseplants, an African violet, and a Christmas cactus. Their familiar presence offers comfort, while caring for them gives her a sense of purpose and motivation to regain strength for returning home.

As we begin unpacking her belongings, we pull out a Sharpie. Nothing goes into the drawers without a label—her first initial and last name. Every shirt, every pair of underwear, even her hairbrush is marked, just as I once did when I sent my kids off to summer camp.

Though the facility assures me that each resident's laundry is washed separately, labeling is still encouraged because things have a way of disappearing.

Along with clothing, the move-in list includes essentials like toiletries and personal items. For Mom, this means non-allergenic arthritic cream, denture wash, and her favorite sweatshirt. Depending on the individual, families may also need to provide incontinence supplies, such as adult diapers or pads.

Ask if the facility takes care of residents' laundry. Some require the family to pick up the laundry, have it cleaned, and returned each week.

A Personal Touch

Wanting to make this transition as smooth as possible and ease my own anxiety about leaving Mom and returning home to Texas, I create a flower arrangement for her room with winter-white branches wrapped in twinkling lights. This small memento stays with her throughout her healthcare journey, serving as both a night light and a quiet reminder of my presence when I can't be with her.

Keeping the Care Staff Coming Back

Whether hosting a house full of teenagers or training adults on the latest software, one thing never fails to draw people in—food. Set out a bowl of candy bars and chips and people swarm. It's a surefire way of being the most popular person in the room.

I apply this same strategy to Mom's rehab stay. Her nightstand drawer is fully stocked with goodies—M&M's, Starbursts, Hershey's Kisses, and Oreos. Word spreads quickly, and by late evening, once all the residents are tucked in for the night, nurses and care partners start trickling in to 'check on Mom.'

She welcomes them with a smile and gestures toward the stash.

"Help yourself," she says.

They stay. They chat.

It's a win-win and a small price to pay to keep eyes on Mom more frequently when we aren't around.

Communicating with the Staff: How to Advocate Effectively for the Patient

As with all 'Mom tasks,' my sister and I divide and conquer. While I focus on setting up her room, Tina tracks down the nurse to review hospital discharge orders and confirm medications. She also ensures the rehab facility has emergency contact information, details for Mom's primary care physician, and her medical directives.

Immediately, Tina notices a disconnect between the hospital's instructions and what we know works for Mom. For one, her blood pressure always runs high. What's considered a "normal" reading for her often alarms medical staff. And timing medications correctly is crucial. Too late, and her numbers spike too early, and she risks dizziness and fainting.

Unlike many, Mom's chronic hypertension isn't rooted in coronary artery disease but instead by anxiety, fear, and deep-seated phobias. With every hospitalization and every new facility, we educate the medical team responsible for her care, reinforcing this vital information.

ADVOCACY IS ESSENTIAL

Fortunately, Mom is fearless about speaking up. She knows every medication she takes and the reasons behind them, a testament to her sharpness. But as her health changes, new prescriptions are introduced, and when she doesn't recognize the pills, her instinct is to resist, leading to conflict with the dispensing nurse.

Be the patient's advocate. Know their medications, understand the reasons behind each prescription, and stay informed on dosing schedules. Ideally, both the patient and their family serve as advocates, holding the medical team accountable, but older adults may not feel comfortable or be able to challenge medical professionals. This means caregivers must ask questions. Double-check everything. Reconfirm that the correct medications are being administered and proper procedures are being followed. This is not just a best practice. It's a patient's right and a caregiver's responsibility.

ALLERGIES

One of the most critical points we emphasize is Mom's extreme sensitivity to medications. While it might take three extra-strength ibuprofens to tackle a migraine for me, a single baby aspirin does the trick for her.

We've seen firsthand how dangerous missteps can be—hives and stage four pressure ulcers form on Mom's legs, causing tissue loss, as well as muscle and tendon damage. And once, a medication misdiagnosis nearly sealed her fate.

PT and OT Demystified:
How Therapy Helps Patients Get Back on Their Feet

After Tina has squared things away with the medical staff, and I've set up Mom's room with a homey touch, we regroup. There's one more stop we need to make—the gym where she will be receiving physical and occupational therapy. Mom's resting in her room; the day has worn her out. She'll see the gym another day.

Tina and I slip through the back gym door, careful not to disrupt sessions in progress. It's an impressive space, and a primary reason we chose this facility.

A therapist, Christopher, steps out from the back office to greet us. "How can I help you?" he asks. We explain that our mom just arrived, and we hand over paperwork from the hospital listing the prescribed exercise and treatment plan she is to begin. Christopher thanks us and says, "Yes, I was just reviewing your mom's admittance chart. I'll stop by and introduce myself to her later today."

> Physical Therapy (PT) is a healthcare discipline focused on improving movement, strength, and overall physical function. It helps individuals recover from injuries, manage chronic conditions, and regain mobility after surgeries or illnesses. A physical therapist works with patients to develop personalized treatment plans that may include exercises, stretches, manual therapy, and specialized techniques like heat or cold therapy. They assist with pain management, balance training, and rehabilitation for conditions such as arthritis, stroke recovery, and sports injuries. Additionally, physical therapists educate patients on injury prevention and lifestyle modifications to enhance long-term well-being. Their goal is to restore independence and improve quality of life through targeted movement-based interventions.

We ask about occupational therapy, and Christopher says that the therapist isn't in at the moment but invites us to look at the OT space. Connected to the gym is a separate room—a replica of a small apartment, complete with a kitchen and bathroom.

> Occupational therapists (OTs) help individuals regain or improve their ability to perform daily activities. They work with people recovering from injuries, managing disabilities, or adjusting to physical, cognitive, or emotional challenges. An OT develops personalized strategies to foster independence, whether that means relearning everyday tasks like dressing and cooking, improving mobility, or adapting environments to better suit their needs.

"I'm not an OT," Christopher says, "but I can tell you the ones here do a great job. I've seen it firsthand."

He reaches for two devices, each hanging from a hook. "This is a grabber," he says, demonstrating how squeezing the handle extends the reach and allows him to grab a towel hanging from a cabinet.

Next, he picks up a second tool. "This is a sock aid, or sock helper. It's designed for people with limited mobility or joint pain to put on socks without bending or straining." He squeezes the flexible metal tube and slides a sock onto it. "If you can't bend over, you just drop this to the floor, slide your foot in, pull the short ropes on either side—and there you have it, your sock is on."

"I'm not sure if your mom will be receiving speech therapy, but we have a speech pathologist here, too."

Speech therapy is a specialized treatment designed to help individuals improve their communication, language, and swallowing abilities. Conducted by speech-language pathologists (SLPs), it addresses a range of disorders, including speech sound difficulties, fluency issues like stuttering, voice disorders, and cognitive-communication challenges. Therapy sessions may involve exercises to strengthen oral muscles, techniques to enhance pronunciation and articulation, and strategies to improve comprehension and expression. For individuals with swallowing difficulties, SLPs provide interventions to ensure safe eating and drinking. Speech therapy benefits people of all ages, from children with developmental delays to adults recovering from strokes or neurological conditions, helping them regain confidence and independence in their daily interactions.

Wrapping Up Rehab Check-In

Satisfied that we've checked everything off our list, we peek into Mom's room one last time before leaving. She's sound asleep.

As we pass through the lobby, we spot Joyce. We thank her and let her know that, as far as we can tell, Mom is all set.

"I have one more question," I say. "Can you clarify the wheelchair situation? Mom doesn't have her own. Does she need one? She also doesn't have a cane or a walker."

"We have equipment she can use while she's here," Joyce reassures me. "Part of the PT and OT evaluations will determine what durable medical equipment she'll need when she's discharged. Depending on the patient, that might mean a wheelchair, a walker, or other adaptive tools. She just got here. Let us work with her, get to know her needs. There's plenty of time to figure all of that out. You ladies have done an excellent job. We'll take good care of her."

Relieved, exhausted and validated, we thank Joyce, say our goodbyes and head home. It's been a long couple of days. A long month. But we did it.

Back at Mom's house, I collapse into bed. Tears spill freely. I'm numb.

And finally, I can return home. I miss my husband. I miss my sons. I miss my dog.

After one last restless night on a rock-hard mattress, I wake up, start packing and tidy up–strip the bed; wash the sheets; clean the bathroom. I also clear out the refrigerator, tossing anything that won't keep until my next visit.

Before heading to the airport, I stop by to see Mom one last time. I'm eager to see how her night went, hopeful she got a good night's rest.

It's mid-morning when I approach her room. The door is partially closed; the lights are off.

Why isn't she up? It's nearly lunchtime.

"Mom," I say, nudging the door open.

"Come in," she answers, her voice thick with annoyance.

"How are you? How'd you sleep?"

"Terrible. The woman next door had her TV blaring all night, and I had to go to the bathroom, but no one came to help me."

Her frustration spills over. She threatens to report them to Medicare, loudly proclaiming her rights.

"The surgery didn't work. I think my hip is still broken," she continues. "The staff is awful. They aren't very personable at all. I try to be friendly, but they're just rude and hateful."

I sigh, knowing this is where she needs to be. I reassure her that things will get better. She just needs to work with the therapists, get stronger and regain muscle strength.

She restarts her tirade, and I interrupt her.

"Mom, I'm sorry. I need to leave. I'm heading home today."

I kiss her forehead, tell her I love her, and step out the door.

Change can be challenging, and adjusting to an unfamiliar environment takes time. Offer support but recognize when it's best to step back and let the transition unfold naturally. Like dropping off a child at school, the initial discomfort is normal. They just need time to settle in and find their footing.

As Tina drives me to the airport, we reflect on everything—what we've endured, what we've accomplished, and what Mom has survived this past month. It's been a lot. But we've survived.

"At least she's settled for now," I say. "I'm not sure how long she'll be there, but from what they said at the hospital, it sounds like at least three weeks."

Tina shakes her head. "Maybe. That's how long Medicare typically covers a rehab stay. It depends on the patient."

I know she's right. But I need to believe Mom is going to stay in rehab, at least for a little while.

I need to believe I can step back into my normal life, even if only temporarily.

Little do I know how short that "little while" will be.

CHAPTER 6

A Broken System

Topics

— Speaking Up with Purpose: Advocating with Impact

— You're Not Alone: Shared Struggles of a Flawed System

— The DME Maze: Navigating Durable
  Medical Equipment Challenges

Navigating Mom's healthcare journey is a crash course in systemic dysfunction. We encountered a fragmented maze of insurance approvals, disconnected medical history from one physician to another and an avalanche of red tape that leaves us overwhelmed and scrambling.

We also learn that staying organized, advocating fiercely, and speaking up when something seems off are essential survival skills. Mom is unable to use the bathroom without help, let alone cook meals or fulfill daily tasks. It's not safe for her to return home alone, at least not yet. But according to 'the system' she's ready to be discharged from rehab, rolled out onto the facility's front porch, overnight bag in hand, blanket across her lap, catching an Uber ride home.

RESUMING MY *OTHER* LIFE

From the moment I got the call that Mom had fallen and had been lying on the floor in her home for four days, I've been riding a relentless wave of emotions. My fight-or-flight response has been in overdrive with shock, fear, panic and frustration. But now, after three long, unpredictable weeks in St. Louis, weeks that felt more like months, I'm finally back home in Texas.

Mom is finally adjusting. She's in a hand-picked rehab facility that my sister and I found in record time. Her meds are stabilized; PT and OT orders are in place; she's safe and set up for success.

Missing Thanksgiving with my husband and sons hurt more than I expected. But I'm happy to be back to them in time to enjoy the festivities leading up to Christmas. I know I'll need to return to St. Louis before the holiday because Medicare only covers up to twenty-one days of rehab, but for now, I can breathe. I can regroup. And I can get a good night's sleep in my own bed.

Resuming life in my home-office, Monday is all about reacclimating to work, clearing out the clutter of neglected emails and finally tackling the meetings I've been dodging. By Tuesday morning, I've hit my stride, kicking things off with a quick staff check-in. It feels good to return to a space where the expectations are clear and the path to success is familiar. Navigating resistant team members and impossible timelines? That's a challenge I know how to meet. The rules make sense here, unlike my role as project manager of Mom's life where I'm still fumbling my way along because there's so much *I know I don't know.*

I glance at my phone, seeing a missed call and voicemail. The number isn't familiar, but the area code is St. Louis. My body tightens instinctively. I brace myself and press play, slipping from fight or flight mode into fight *and* flight mode. *I hope Mom is okay.*

The call is from Joyce, the social worker. Her voice is upbeat, almost celebratory. "Your mom's doing great. She's excelling on the cognitive tests, and she's made solid progress with physical and occupational therapy. We're preparing to discharge her."

Wait. What?! Send her home? She's only been there five days. She's allowed up to twenty-one days of rehab. My mind goes blank. I can't process this. I press end, disconnecting from voicemail, and I immediately call back. Three rings. The receptionist answers. I interrupt her. "Can I speak to Joyce, please?"

After a brief hold, Joyce picks up.

"Joyce, this is Marlene's daughter," I say.

"Oh, I just left you a voice--"

"I know. That's why I'm calling." My voice is sharp. "She's only been there a few days. She has up to twenty-one days."

Joyce doesn't flinch. Her tone matches mine. "I said rehab could take up to twenty-one days. But your mom's doing so well, she's ready to go home."

"She can't go home," I say firmly. "I don't live there. I just flew back to Texas. She has nowhere to go. She lives alone, and I'm almost certain she's not walking unassisted... is she?"

"Well, no," Joyce replies, "but she's doing well."

"She's not going home," I snap. "I'll catch a flight and be back tomorrow. We need to meet."

I don't wait for agreement. "My sister and I will be at your facility at one o'clock. I want a meeting—with you, the PT, the OT, and anyone else involved in her care."

So much for my self-proclaimed lessons on relationship building and 'playing nice.'

> Medicare Part A (Hospital Insurance) covers medically necessary care in an inpatient rehabilitation facility (IRF) for acute care rehabilitation for patients who have suffered a stroke, a traumatic injury or are recovering from a major surgery. To qualify, a physician must certify a medical condition requiring intensive rehabilitation, continued medical supervision, and coordinated care from your doctors, other health care providers, and therapists. In most cases, the patient pays nothing for days one through twenty in a benefit period after the Part A deductible is met. Then, between days twenty-one and one hundred of the benefit period, a per-day charge set by Medicare is the responsibility of the patient.

> **Resource:** Inpatient Rehabilitation Facility (IRF)
> Reference Booklet (https://www.cms.gov/files/document/
> inpatientrehabilitationfacilityrefbooklet2pdf)

Speaking Up with Purpose: Advocating with Impact

I return the next day, and Tina and I meet with Mom's care team. It has only been six days since she entered rehab, and we are stunned that they're already recommending discharge. She still relies heavily on her wheelchair and can only manage short distances with a walker, neither of which can be done without help.

Once again, we find ourselves repeating what we told the hospital social worker just days earlier: Mom lives alone. She's not ready to return home. She needs more time. Time to rebuild strength, regain mobility, and reestablish a level of independence.

After a tense back-and-forth exchange, the team concedes. While adhering to Medicare requirements, the team agrees that Mom can benefit from a little more time in rehab. They tell us it may not be the full twenty-one days, but we are thankful to have secured at least another week or two.

Relief washes over me. We have time to regroup, reassess, and figure out our next move.

Do not be passive or overly accommodating. Championing the patient's needs often means diplomatically pushing back, asking hard questions, and challenging assumptions. Healthcare teams may base their recommendations on a mix of legal constraints, precedent, financial pressures, and even interpersonal dynamics. But as the voice of the patient, challenge decisions. If something feels off, speak up. Silence serves no one.

Negotiating to extend Mom's rehab stay is not our last clash with the facility. Despite her medical chart clearly listing severe medication sensitivities and documented allergies, and without notifying Tina or me, Mom is prescribed steroids for a minor infection, resulting in a fever. The staff wants to send her back to the hospital, but we push back.

"No! She doesn't need *another* hospital admission. She needs Tylenol and Benadryl" we insist. The facility refuses to administer either. It is Saturday and no doctor's orders are on file, so the staff won't break protocol.

Our solution? I make a quick trip to the nearest CVS, buy a bottle of Tylenol, return to the facility, and hand Mom two pills with a cup of water. Within an hour, her low-grade fever breaks, and she starts feeling herself again.

Be aware that some medications can have counter-effects when taken together, so consult a physician for guidance. If you know what works for the patient, request doctor's orders for over the counter (OTC) medications as needed, otherwise referred to as PRN (pro re nata).

Everyone Has a Story

Our run-in with the hospital social worker and the figurative threat of Mom being left like a potted plant on the porch of the rehab facility are just a few examples of cracks in the disjointed medical system. Over the coming months and years, we learn that anyone caring for aging parents has a 'you won't believe what happened to us' story.

From Texas to Missouri, friends and colleagues share their own tales— some heartbreaking, some infuriating—all pointing to the same truth: the system is broken. Here are just a few examples.

You're Not Alone: Shared Struggles of a Flawed System

Renee shares a story about transferring her mother from one rehab facility to another and the challenges she faced.

My mom was in a rehab hospital following a car accident. I loved the facility. It was a clean, uplifting, positive environment with a great gym. Mom met some nice people. She did okay for the first two weeks, but she reached a point where she wasn't improving and the therapy was too intense for her, so we needed to move her.

I was back to the drawing board. I found another place, and we packed her up and off she went. The facility she moved into was nice, but I still felt the need to visit her daily. She had complications from her accident, and changing medical dressings of her open wounds wasn't part of the services the rehab center provided. I'm not sure why. She needed a bandage changed. They should have been able to do that.

Anyway, this new rehab facility worked better for her. The rehab exercises weren't as intense, and the center operated at a slower pace.

The problem is that the system isn't set up for you to move from one rehab facility to another. Apparently, the new place didn't get an approval ahead of time, so several months later, long after Mom was released, we got a bill for four-thousand dollars.

I called Medicare, and after what felt like hours on hold, I finally got through to a person. I explained the situation, and they read the standard customer service script, "I'm sorry. It is our policy that authorization must be obtained before entering a rehabilitation facility."

"We did get the pre-authorization. We just needed to move her. The first place wasn't working out for her," I explained.

Frustrated and worn down after multiple phone calls and countless repetitions of the same story, I gave up. I just threw my hands up and paid the bill. I wasn't going to win this battle. No matter how many times I tried explaining how the series of events unfolded.

HANGING OUT IN THE HALLWAY

Here's an excerpt from Mark. His dad had knee surgery that resulted in complications. When Mark's dad went into rehab, he needed both heart and knee rehabilitation exercises. But the challenges set in before they ever step foot into his dad's room.

> My dad went in for routine knee surgery. He had complications that resulted in knee rehabilitation and heart rehab. The hospital social worker set everything up, and they arranged transportation for Dad from the hospital to the rehab facility. Assuming we had time before the transfer, we left the hospital and stopped for dinner before the driver picked him up. When we got to rehab, we asked what room Dad was in, and they said, "We don't have any space right now. He doesn't have a room assigned yet." They pointed and said, "He's down that hallway."
>
> Sure enough, Dad was near the end of the hall up against the wall. He was in a wheelchair with his leg elevated. He hadn't eaten. We didn't know if he had taken his meds, and we had no idea how long he'd be without a room assignment.
>
> My wife stepped in. "This is ridiculous. He needs a room, and he needs dinner." She worked her magic and talked to the right people. They told us we could wheel him down to the cafeteria so he could eat dinner while we waited for space to open. Finally, at 10 p.m., he was assigned a room. We got him settled and left. If we hadn't gone by to check on him, who knows how long he would have sat in that hall.

The DME Maze: Navigating Durable Medical Equipment Challenges

It's common for breaks in the system to surface around durable medical equipment—wheelchairs, walkers, hospital beds. We have our own, *you won't believe our story*, experience when trying to secure a wheelchair for Mom.

Several years into Mom's healthcare journey, when she was living in a long-term care facility, the rental wheelchair she'd been using was no longer working. It didn't fit her body properly, compressing her spine and intensifying her pain.

We reached out to a wheelchair specialist for a solution. They sent over a physical therapist and a medical equipment rep to fit Mom for a custom chair. They took custom measurements and designed a chair tailored just for her.

The catch: We're told Medicare likely won't cover the cost. Why? Because Mom is living in a private-pay, long-term care facility, and the 'rules' say that the facility should provide the equipment. For rehab in a facility, this is true. For a private-pay resident permanently living in a facility, this is not true. The facility is Mom's 'home' address.

Our options are limited:

1. Have the wheelchair delivered to my sister's permanent address, but that won't work, since Mom needs to be present for final adjustments.

2. Pay out of pocket without filing through Medicare, a seven-thousand-dollar expense.

3. Hope the supplier can advocate on Mom's behalf to get Medicare to approve the chair.

Option three works. The equipment supplier bills Medicare, lobbies on Mom's behalf, and she receives a custom-built wheelchair that improves her range of motion, posture and overall quality of life, reducing pain in her spine. Success.

But the story doesn't end there. After Mom's passing, no longer needing the wheelchair, I dropped it off at a resale shop specializing in durable medical equipment. A week later, I got a call from the wheelchair supplier asking for the chair back.

"What? I don't have it anymore."

That's when I learn she hadn't even owned the chair. It was a rental. I had unknowingly donated a seven-thousand-dollar piece of equipment, and if I couldn't get it back, we'd be on the hook for the full cost—a nearly ten-thousand-dollar chair for a woman who was no longer alive.

Thankfully, I was able to coordinate with the resale shop, the supplier sent a driver to retrieve the wheelchair, and the crisis was averted.

Here's yet another—durable medical equipment—broken system story. This one is from Cindy, who needed to find a creative alternative for getting her mom, Betty, a much-needed hospital bed in the long-term care facility where she lived.

My mom, Betty, had an episode at her assisted living facility. She was eating dinner when she aspirated, choking on her food and obstructing her airway. The staff jumped into action, calming her down, helping her swallow, and getting her breathing normally again, but the incident shook her. While aspiration is common among older adults, it was new for my mom and for us.

A few days later, she was taken to the hospital—her vitals were off and she was confused, so she was admitted for observation. While she was there, we learned that she could not return to assisted living; her needs had progressed beyond what they could safely manage. Suddenly, we were searching for a new place, and we eventually found a longterm care facility.

After only a few weeks in her new environment, her health continued declining requiring two people to lift and transfer her into and out of her bed. The staff recommended we get her a hospital bed to replace the standard facility-provided bed. The challenge was that Medicare refused to cover it unless she was on hospice. We worked with a hospice coordinator, but we still couldn't secure a bed for her.

> Frustrated but undeterred, we pivoted. A home health company connected us with a family who had recently purchased a hospital bed that had never been used. The bed had been delivered just before the family member who needed it was hospitalized and never returned home. The family couldn't return it, and they no longer needed it, so they gave it to us—refusing any payment. Our plan is to pay it forward and donate it to another family when my mom no longer needs it.

Regardless of the story, everyone eventually collides with the broken healthcare system. It's a frustrating, overwhelming, and exhausting experience, full of twists, turns, and resistance. Caring for an aging parent is already mentally and emotionally demanding; layering on the burden of navigating a disjointed system with inconsistent processes and fragmented information makes it even harder.

Take good notes. Keep a running chronology of events as they unfold. Advocate fiercely for your loved one and question decisions made by staff and medical professionals. Be respectful, but courageous. Only the care team and the patient truly understand the full story. The professionals brought in along the way see only a snapshot moment in time of their journey.

CHAPTER 7

Respite Care—Mom's Stop Off Before Returning Home

Topics

— Respite Care 101: What It Is and When to Use It

— Choosing Respite Care: What to Look for
and Questions to Ask

— Settling In at Respite Care: It's Still Not Home

The good news is that Mom's rehab extension was approved. Medicare granted her the full twenty-one days, which gives us the time to figure out where we go from here. While she's stronger, she's not ready to return home and pick up where she left off. She still needs additional support. The question is, now that rehab is ending, what's next? Once again, I find myself navigating unfamiliar territory and facing another steep learning curve.

Since *I don't know what I don't know* about Mom's recovery journey, I'm challenged once again trying to navigate unfamiliar terrain. It feels like a never-ending "do-loop": every time I tackle one major milestone, another unknown challenge pops up.

The unfortunate *fortunate* thing I learn over the coming years is that I can apply and reapply newly learned skills with each fall. For instance, like many her age, Mom becomes a frequent faller. One study by UT

Austin's College of Liberal Arts found that thirty-four percent of adults aged seventy and older experienced two or more falls within a three-year period.

Geriatric specialists warn me that Mom will likely fall again, and dismissively I think, 'No, not my mom. She's strong and fit. I don't see her being a statistic. Boy, am I wrong. Listen and learn from the professionals. Believe what they say. Don't bury your head in the sand and think not us. Have a plan. Consider options. Talk with your aging parent and siblings about strategies and 'what if' scenarios. Mom's first fall may not be grounds for putting a for-sale sign in her front yard, but it may be a pivotal moment to begin having difficult conversations.

Respite Care 101: What It Is and When to Use It

Mom reaches the end of her stay in rehab, but she's not yet able to return home and live by herself. She still needs physical and occupational therapy; she can't prepare meals or stand for extended periods; and she isn't able to drive. Returning to her home alone isn't an option. We need another choice. The rehab staff recommends respite care.

Respite care offers short-term, temporary support for individuals with disabilities, chronic illnesses, or other ongoing needs, allowing their family or primary caregivers a much-needed break. This relief gives caregivers the opportunity to rest, address personal matters, or focus on other aspects of their lives.

This is exactly our situation. From the moment I got the call that Mom had fallen and was rushed to the hospital, I've been by her side, living in her home for weeks, returning to Texas briefly, then flying back to St. Louis. The constant back-and-forth is taking a toll. I feel exhausted, overwhelmed, and frustrated. With Christmas just days away, I long to be home in Texas with my husband and sons, but I'm struggling to balance my own needs with Mom's care.

'Clear your head. Get focused. You need a plan,' I tell myself. To have any hope of spending the holiday back home, I need to find a place where Mom can continue recovering. So, I begin researching respite care options.

In my search, I come across The National Institute of Aging website (https://www.nia.nih.gov/health/what-respite-care), which offers resources on paying for respite services, support systems and more. Helpful resources to search include:

- State Respite Registries
- State Respite Coalitions
- State Lifespan Respite Programs
- National Family Caregiver Support Program
- Respite for Veterans
- Adult Day Care Centers

I discover that respite care services are typically billed on an hourly or length-of-stay basis, whether for a few hours or several days or weeks. Unfortunately, most insurance plans do not cover these costs, meaning any expenses not covered by insurance or other funding sources will be your responsibility.

CREATE A LIST OF PLACES TO VISIT

With a clearer understanding of what respite care is, I begin my search, narrowing results by reviewing online feedback, researching safety concerns, and considering proximity to both Mom's house and my sister's.

Despite specifying 'near me,' some facilities appear forty-five minutes to an hour away—distances that simply won't work for us. Over the past several weeks, juggling Mom's hospitalization and rehab has reinforced how crucial location is. I've made countless trips back and forth, trying to meet Mom's needs while balancing my professional responsibilities.

One place touts an onsite therapy dog that interacts with the residents. I 'star' this option. Mom loves dogs, and this might be a great way to get her buy-in.

Another facility prioritizes social and physical well-being, featuring an onsite gym with regularly scheduled Silver Sneakers exercise classes. Since staying active is key to maintaining independence, this location also earns a spot on my list.

The third facility emphasizes staff development, ensuring team members receive specialized training in the psychology of aging. While not all locations have a full-time geriatric psychologist on staff, having well-trained caregivers who understand the challenges older adults face, especially for someone like Mom, who experiences high anxiety and chronic phobias, can make a meaningful difference in her comfort and care.

> Geriatric psychologists, also known as geropsychologists, specialize in the mental health needs of older adults, playing a vital role in senior living facilities. They provide tailored services, including diagnosis, treatment, and counseling for conditions such as depression, anxiety, dementia, and other age-related mental health challenges.

Staff in senior living facilities undergo specialized training based on state and facility requirements, often including coursework in geriatrics, the study of social, psychological, and biological aspects of aging. This training equips them to understand and address residents' unique needs.

Dementia is prevalent among older adults, and staff often receive specialized instruction on managing behavioral changes, fostering a safe and supportive environment, and communicating effectively with those affected. Falls also pose a serious risk, and staff are trained in prevention techniques, such as assessing risk factors, creating a secure environment, and implementing strategies to minimize fall-related incidents.

Having staff who understand the emotional and psychological needs of geriatric residents is important, especially since Mom was confused and showed potential signs of dementia when she was admitted to the hospital.

An alternative to respite care in a facility is hiring in-home caregivers. With Mom's circumstances, we would have needed help with continuous medication management; nightly trips to the bathroom; coordinating PT and OT; and meal preparation. Since respite care and aging in place (meaning a loved one stays in their own home) are new concepts for me, and time is limited for making next-step decisions, we ultimately opt to stick with only exploring facility-based respite care options.

Practical Alternatives to Paid Respite Care

- **Adult Day Programs:** Some community centers, churches, or nonprofits offer low-cost or slidingscale adult day services where seniors can spend time safely while caregivers rest or work.

- **Community and FaithBased Resources:** Local organizations often provide volunteer companions, meal delivery, or short-term caregiving support. These can be free or donation based.

- **Family and Friends Rotation:** Coordinating with siblings, extended family, or trusted friends to share caregiving duties. Even a few-hour break can provide meaningful respite without financial cost.

- **In Home Support Services:** Some municipalities or nonprofits offer visiting aides or homemaker services at reduced rates, especially for seniors with limited income.

- **Government Programs:** Medicaid (in the U.S.) and similar programs in other countries may cover limited respite or home health services if your parent qualifies.

Choosing Respite Care: What to Look for and Questions to Ask

QUESTIONS TO ASK WHEN VISITING RESPITE CARE FACILITIES

When compiling a list of respite care facilities and preparing for visits, it's wise to have a set of questions ready. After visiting multiple locations, details can sometimes blur together, making it difficult to remember which facility provided which information. To stay organized, consider asking the following ten questions, and add others that are important:

1. Do staff members undergo background checks?

2. What safety measures are in place?

3. Is the facility equipped with a monitored security system?

4. Are staff required to hold specific licenses and certifications?

5. What are the costs, and when are payments due?

6. How does the facility handle emergencies, whether it's a resident's medical issue or natural disasters like tornadoes?

7. Can I speak with residents to hear about their experiences at the facility?

8. What is the staff-to-resident ratio?

9. How do you address specific concerns raised in online reviews?

10. What services are included in respite care, and what additional offerings are not covered?

This list serves as a solid foundation for evaluating each facility's quality and suitability. Adding personalized questions based on priorities can help ensure the best fit.

Hoping my research and short-listing of three facilities will help me avoid less than ideal options, I pull into the parking lot of the first one. It's a two-story brick building, and it made my shortlist because it offers regularly scheduled exercise classes—an important feature for Mom. She loves staying active, and being active isn't just about staying strong; it's her preferred way to heal versus taking medication.

Despite the picturesque, wooded surroundings, the facility itself feels outdated, worn, and uninviting. The tour guide, a resident filling in because they are shorthanded, offers insight that confirms my instincts. When I ask about the advertised exercise classes, she responds, "Oh, we don't do that anymore. I've been here for over a year, and we've never had anything like that."

I quickly wrap up my tour. There's no need for further questions. It's clear this isn't the right place. Time to check out the next option on my list.

The second stop isn't much better. This location is clean, organized and more professional than the last, but it, too, has problems. As I enter the lobby, the woman at the desk hands me a clipboard with forms and barks, "Fill these out."

The top portion is standard demographic info—Mom's name, date of birth, and so on, but the next section brings me pause. It is about Mom's financial solvency. Questions include: How much liquidity does she have? What portion is available from checking and savings accounts versus retirement accounts? Another section wants me to state her net worth and whether she owns a home. If so, what is the value, and is there an outstanding mortgage?

I am not comfortable with this. I haven't even had a tour yet, and they want a full financial disclosure? I write 'available upon request' in the blanks and return the incomplete forms to the receptionist, telling her I would rather not provide the private information as I'm just here for a tour.

"No problem," she says. "Let's get started."

Our first stop is the 'gym,' a converted office space with a large exercise ball, some resistance bands and a few hand weights. We make a quick pass through the dining hall, and I politely thank her and make my way towards the front door. There's no need wasting her time or mine. This place isn't right for Mom either.

Over time, I grow to understand the importance of the financial viability questionnaire. While not relevant to respite care, its questions are crucial for those seeking long-term care. In some cases, elders with enough funds to cover three years at a facility may become eligible for subsidized housing, such as Medicaid.

In one instance, I witnessed firsthand the heartbreaking reality of a resident in a long-term care facility who depleted her savings and was forced to leave her home. She made friends and loved where she was living, but she ran out of money. She left in tears, and the experience was devastating for her. Assisted living and long-term care are often funded out-of-pocket. A clear understanding of an elder's financial situation helps both the resident and the facility plan ahead.

My third stop of the day is to the facility with the dog—a black lab that wanders around keeping the residents' company. I'm most excited about this visit and hope it lives up to the marketing hype on the website. This place looks more like a luxury hotel than a retirement community. I remind myself, *Don't let beauty cloud your judgment. This is about elder care, staff ratios and whether it is a good, safe fit for Mom.*

I meet Brandy, the director of admissions. She is professional, warm, and immediately puts me at ease. As we talk, I share Mom's journey over the past several weeks, and unexpectedly, emotion overtakes me. Tears fill my eyes. My voice falters. I barely know this woman, yet here I am, breaking down in front of her. *What's wrong with me? I am not usually a crier.* But the weight of everything—the decisions, the uncertainty, the exhaustion—comes rushing in all at once.

Brandy doesn't flinch. She slides a box of tissues toward me and reassures me that what I'm feeling is completely normal. Her kindness steadies me, and soon, our conversation flows. We talk not just about Mom but about our families, our husbands, our kids, our lives. In that moment, I feel truly seen and supported. Our conversation shifts to details about the facility, the amenities they offer and the varying levels of care available from independent living to assisted living to memory care, and the part I'm most interested in, respite care.

Keep a record of all the people you meet along the way. Years after my initial visit, I reached out to Brandy when I once again needed help navigating Mom's living arrangements. I sent her a quick text, and she responded immediately. Though she had since moved out of state, she didn't hesitate to offer support, providing me with a local point of contact in St. Louis who could assist.

We tour the facility, stopping by the game room where residents are putting together a puzzle. And wandering the hallways, as promised, is the infamous black lab who greets me with a gentle nudge of her cold nose and a friendly wag of her tail, instantly winning me over.

I love everything about this place, but before I get too attached, I ask, "Do you have respite space available? Mom is about to be discharged from rehab, and we need to move her within the next three days."

Brandy confirms that, yes, the respite room should be available, as the resident in the space is expected to be moving out within the next few days. Perfect. Our last stop on the tour is a visit to the respite room model. This is an exact replica of the room where Mom will be staying. It is beautiful. Matching drapes and comforter, a small kitchenette with a sink and cabinets, and a mahogany chest of drawers that doubles as a TV stand.

Research and have options lined up ahead of time. Have a first, second and third choice of places where you are comfortable with your aging parent staying because decisions and next steps happen fast and often with little warning. One day, a facility is at capacity and the next day, they have open rooms. Elder care and facility availability is a fluid environment, and our fortunate experience is that everything works out. So, plan, coordinate and strategize in advance, and then exercise patience as things unfold in real-time.

Unable to contain myself, I blurt out, "I'll take it." Catching myself, I quickly qualify my commitment with, "But I guess I need to understand how much it will cost, what's included, and I'll also need my sister to visit as we are making these decisions together."

SIGNING THE CONTRACT FOR RESPITE CARE

I plan a return visit with Tina so we can review the contract, pay the deposit, and get things rolling. Time is of the essence.

Some contract terms resemble those found in an apartment rental agreement, but there are key differences. For instance, this facility partners with a designated pharmacy, and its contract requires that all medications are dispensed in blister pack containers. (Think of the individually sealed bubbles that over-the-counter cold medicine often comes in.) These packs help prevent pills from going missing while also providing staff with a clear, visual indicator of when a patient has received their medication.

We initially want to continue using Mom's long-standing mail-order pharmacy, as her supplemental insurance covers much of the cost, keeping her out-of-pocket expenses low. Ultimately, we give in and agree to use the facility's affiliated pharmacy with the understanding that, if her costs turn out to be higher than mail order, we reserve the right to revisit the agreement.

In the end, the pharmacy costs are the same, but we later discover that the partnership between the pharmacy and the facility isn't solely about convenience; there are partial stakeholder ownerships in both businesses.

Read the fine print when signing a contract. Confirm if there are stipulations around whether a specific pharmacy is used, and whether you can provide medication refills from an alternative provider. Also, are you required to give notice when ending the contract? Like short-term rental agreements, is there a required security deposit and, if so, is it reimbursed when the resident moves out?

Settling In at Respite Care: It's Still Not Home

As promised, the respite room is spotless and ready for us on Saturday, giving us time to add a few personal touches before Mom's Monday arrival. Everything is falling into place, and I am relieved I'll be able to get her settled, fly home to Texas, and be with my husband and sons before Christmas.

Just like the model room, Mom's space features a twin bed, a big-screen TV, and a kitchenette with a mini fridge. She has a private bathroom, which we stock with fresh towels and toiletries. We remake the bed with crisp new sheets and a fresh pillow, a small way of pampering her that I soon realize is entirely mine—not Mom's. She feels most at home with threadbare linens and a rock-hard mattress, reinforced with a piece of plywood for extra firmness. Comfort, to her, is familiarity, not luxury. No matter how much I encourage her to indulge, she resists.

Years later, I come to understand—her simpler lifestyle isn't about rejecting comfort but embracing what she's always known. And inversely, I continue reframing the message in my life, choosing self-care as a vital practice for my own mental health.

To make her stay more comfortable, we add a mini microwave and bring her coffee maker from home, ensuring she won't have to leave her room for her morning cup of joe. Another familiar touch finds its way into her space—a tabletop statue of three puppies holding a 'Welcome' sign, a long-time fixture in Mom's kitchen.

Bringing a little holiday warmth to the room, we hang a Christmas wreath on the door and decorate with festive pieces from Mom's basement. *She'll love it. I'm sure.*

We make one final touch before the big reveal. Tina and I track down a local photo studio for a long-overdue sibling picture. The last time we posed together was in elementary school, when Mom dressed us in matching tartan jumpers and white peasant blouses.

For this photoshoot, we wear purple, Mom's favorite color, and bring our best adult selves to the shoot—no longer a prepubescent teen nor a toothless, frizzy-haired kid. Despite the challenges we've faced these past weeks, carving out time for this special memory feels deeply meaningful.

When the session wraps up, Tina and I hug a little tighter than usual, sensing, though not fully knowing, that Mom's first stop in respite care won't be her last.

Mom's Arrival

With everything in place, the much-anticipated Monday arrives. I meet Mom at the rehab center, gather her belongings, and wheel her to the front portico where her minivan awaits. She still needs assistance walking, but with support, she stands and carefully maneuvers herself into the passenger seat. Once she's buckled in, we set off for her new temporary home away from home, respite care.

In true Mom fashion, her conversation bounces between frustration over traffic and relief at finally getting some fresh air. "It's so good to be out of that place," she says.

I reassure her. "You're going to love this new place. It's warm, welcoming, and even has a dog."

Her expression shifts. "New place? Wait. I thought I was going home."

Clenching my teeth, steadying my patience, I say, "Not yet, Mom. You are getting stronger, but you need a little more time to recover."

She's unconvinced. "Christopher, the therapist, said I was doing great! I worked harder than anyone, so I can go home. I don't need to be in another one of those places."

This isn't going the way I'd hoped. What should have been a smooth, positive transition is quickly unraveling. I redirect the conversation, shifting to the Christmas presents I've bought for the kids. It distracts her temporarily.

When we arrive, the facility staff is waiting, greeting Mom with love and compassion. They help her out of the van and into a wheelchair. She delivers a passive-aggressive remark, and out of her line of sight, the assisting nurse catches my exasperated expression. We exchange a knowing smile.

Once inside, I take control of the wheelchair, guiding Mom toward her room. As much as I want to showcase the amenities, I know the best approach is to first help her settle into the space, giving her time to adjust. Her mood is not ideal for first impressions with the staff or other residents.

Tina is waiting in the room, ready to welcome her. She points out the puppy statue and the familiar touches from home—small details blended seamlessly with the facility's décor. But Mom remains resistant, defensive, and irritated.

We highlight the positives: her private bathroom, her own coffee maker—but nothing seems to break through her frustration. Finally, Tina picks up the framed photo of the two of us. "Look, Mom," she says, "Merry Christmas. We had this made for you."

Mom's face softens. Tears well in her eyes. "Oh. This is beautiful. Thank you," she whispers. Her voice breaks. With Mom now in a better place, we take her on a quick tour, and the staff introduces her to her tablemates. Dinner service is beginning.

The next morning, I stop by one last time before heading to the airport.

Finally, I can exhale and head home to my family in Texas. I remind myself that I've respectfully and lovingly taken care of Mom. She's in a safe, beautiful place where she can continue recovering. I'll be back soon.

CHRISTMAS EVE

Mid-afternoon on Christmas Eve, the world quiets. Stores close, families gather, and a familiar, peaceful tone blankets the evening—a feeling I've recognized every year since I was young. The familiarity of that feeling settles a peace in my heart that I haven't felt in a while.

But, as we are getting ready for church, my phone rings. The caller ID flashes the name of Mom's facility, and the anxiousness I feel is instant.

I answer. Silence. Then, there is a soft, staggered crying on the other end.

"Mom, breathe. Calm down so I can understand you."

She inhales, exhales. The crying continues, but her words are clearer now.

"I'm sad. I'm lonely. It's Christmas. I want to go home. Please don't make me stay here. Please come get me," she says between gasps of crying.

And just like that, my Christmas cheer is gone. I'm sad. I'm crying. I feel awful.

This is my mom. What am I doing to her?

I try to reassure her. "Mom, you need to be where you are. I'm in Texas, and I can't come right now. It's Christmas Eve."

I tell her how much we love her. We pass the phone around, each family member wishing her a Merry Christmas. By the time the phone returns to me, she sounds steadier.

She apologizes. "I'm so sorry for ruining your Christmas."

"Mom, you haven't ruined anything. We're just happy to hear your voice."

I pivot. "How about I call you tomorrow while the boys open their gifts? You can be part of Christmas morning, even from afar."

A pause. Then, quietly: "I'd like that very much."

"I love you, Mom. Merry Christmas. I'll call you tomorrow."

Caring for an aging parent is hard. We do our best—researching, gathering information, consulting experts, weighing options, making decisions, and hoping they're the right ones. Over the months and years that follow, repeated experiences help us navigate the journey with a little more confidence. But no matter how informed we become, each phase brings new challenges.

Balancing Mom's needs, my own, my family's, and keeping the peace with Tina often feels overwhelming. But, if I approach the process with respect, logic and empathy while keeping Mom's health and safety top of mind, I'm making the best decisions possible with the information available.

Not every decision will be perfect. There may be moments when adjustments are necessary. But if we remain committed to doing the right thing, motivated by love and compassion, we are on the right path.

CHAPTER 8

Work Accommodations and Carving Out a Place of My Own at Mom's

Topics

— Wearing Two Hats: Mom's Care Team
and Working Professional

— Carving Out My Own Space: Adapting Mom's Home
to Support My Needs

— Getting Stuff Done: Creating a Remote Office
That Works

— Setting Boundaries: Sharing Space
and Honoring Our Differences

No matter the distance—across town or across the country—family caregivers often find themselves spending nights, or even extended visits, in their parent's home. I learned practical, easy-to-implement techniques to help create a sense of stability in an otherwise unpredictable situation, including key insights regarding communicating with work colleagues and leadership about my situation and my new role as caregiver for a family member, negotiating accommodations such as flexible hours, remote work options, or Family Medical Leave Act (FMLA) time, and carving out a personal space in Mom's home, a designated area that offers comfort, familiarity, and a moment of respite.

Wearing Two Hats: Mom's Care Team and Working Professional

Mom's house isn't like mine. We shop differently, stock groceries differently, and do laundry differently. We just live differently, so staying at her house is never truly comfortable. What starts as a few nights has stretched into weeks and now months and eventually multiple years of overnight visits. I haven't replaced the mattress yet, though I'm close. I've bought new sheets, pillows, and a blanket to make it feel more like home, but the rock-hard thirty-year-old mattress still makes for a restless night.

As Mom's health declines and regular trips to St. Louis become part of my routine, it becomes clear: I need to make her house more livable for both of us. Comfort matters, especially when caregiving becomes a long-term commitment.

Beyond merging my adult life into Mom's, balancing work responsibilities adds yet another layer of complexity. The strain of managing both professional and personal demands takes a toll on my mental and physical health. Whether caring for toddlers, school-age children, or aging parents, sustaining the illusion of being the perfectly "put-together" professional is exhausting.

Work-life balance looks different for everyone, but in the context of elder care, it often includes last-minute doctor's appointments, unexpected ER visits following a fall and emotionally charged family meetings to reassess care plans. Regardless of proximity, whether living nearby or traveling from out of town, support from the workplace may be needed. Options might include negotiating remote work arrangements, adjusting schedules, or requesting flexible hours to meet the shifting needs of an aging parent's care team.

COMMUNICATION AND WORK ACCOMMODATIONS

While today's work environment may offer more flexibility, clear communication with leadership and a solid understanding of workplace policies can help ease the mental strain of juggling multiple responsibilities. These conversations lay the groundwork for realistic expectations and much needed support.

The Family and Medical Leave Act (FMLA) might be the professional relief needed to help get things settled in the next phase of an aging parent's journey. FMLA provides eligible employees with up to twelve workweeks of unpaid, job-protected leave within a twelve-month period for qualifying family or medical reasons, such as caring for a seriously ill family member. During this leave, employers are required to maintain group health insurance coverage as if the employee were actively working.

Eligibility requires at least twelve months of employment with the current employer and a minimum of 1,250 hours worked in the preceding year.

Most of all, don't feel the need to manage all the competing demands alone. A conversation with a supervisor, a meeting with human resources, or outreach to an employee assistance program can help clarify available support and resources.

> *Communicate with your boss, peers, direct reports and human resource team so they can support you and have a better understanding when you inadvertently miss a meeting or slip on a deadline because you are caring for an aging parent.*

ESCAPE HATCH—HAVING A CAR TO DRIVE

One non-negotiable during stays at Mom's house is access to a car. Whether it's a quick trip to the store or a quiet moment parked in the driveway, having a vehicle nearby helps preserve a sense of sanity. Renting a car at the airport has worked in the past, but regular flights from Texas to St. Louis make that an increasingly expensive option.

Mom and I quickly deduce that driving her minivan while I'm in town makes the most sense. As her health declines, she drives less often, and the van sits idle most days. Having my own transportation provides freedom and independence, and a perfect escape for days when I need to step away.

A lesson I learn the hard way: cars that sit unused need a little extra care. Connecting the van to a trickle charger keeps the battery from draining and ensures it's ready to go when I need it.

*A trickle charger delivers a low, steady current to maintain
a fully charged battery. It's especially useful for vehicles that
remain parked for extended periods, like those stored in garages
or used only occasionally.*

Carving Out My Own Space: Adapting Mom's Home to Support My Needs

To maintain normalcy and to bring a bit of 'me' to Mom's house, I start with a trip to the local beauty supply store, stocking the bathroom with full-size bottles of my favorite shampoo and conditioner instead of constantly refilling travel-size containers. I add makeup and skincare products to my basket, along with a hair dryer and curling iron.

Whether traveling in from out of state or just packing an overnight bag for a stay across town, stocking Mom's house with essentials removes the hassle of remembering what to pack each time. No more scrambling to remember toothpaste, pajamas, or phone chargers. Fewer don't-forget items means less stress, less mental clutter and a lighter travel bag.

One unmistakable difference between Mom's house and mine: the linens. Specifically, the bath towels. Her towels are paper-thin, more like oversized hand towels than anything meant to dry a full-grown body. Most were wedding shower gifts from fifty years ago.

There is one exception, a single set of plush, full-sized towels, a Christmas gift from a few years ago that remain unused. Mom's rationale, "They're too nice to use, too big for my body, and they don't absorb enough water." This set has become unofficially mine. At the end of each visit, I launder the set and return it to *my* closet shelf for the next time.

*Stocking mom's house with everyday essentials you use at home
eases the stress of packing for overnight stays and helps maintain
a sense of normalcy in an otherwise disruptive situation.*

LAUNDRY AT MOM'S

Laundry is yet another area where Mom and I don't see eye to eye. She insists on buying thin, watery detergent, refusing to splurge on name brands because "They're all the same." I beg to differ. She also hates fabric softener, a must-have in every load I do at my own home. To keep the peace, I stock my own supplies, quality detergent, fabric softener, and color-safe bleach, right next to hers.

Since Mom refuses to sleep in the primary bedroom of her own home because Dad slept there before he died, I make this space my sanctuary. I sleep in the bed and use the ensuite bathroom. Each visit, before I head back home, I make sure the trash is empty, my personal items are tucked away, and the sinks and shower are tidy. To accommodate my quick-good-enough cleaning, I have a bottle of all-purpose cleaner and Lysol wipes in the bathroom cabinet. This, in Mom's words, "half-hearted cleaning attempt is a disgrace." If I don't start with a bucket of Pine-Sol, blue Comet powder in the toilet, and vinegar and water in a spray bottle for the mirror, I haven't cleaned the bathroom.

STOCKING THE PANTRY

It's frustrating enough in my own home when I open and close the refrigerator three times, searching for the perfect snack, only to find a bag of grapes, a container of yogurt, and a protein drink staring back at me. And no matter how many times I check, there's still no ooey-gooey treat. This same open and close the refrigerator multiple times routine at Mom's house is even worse—no grapes, no yogurt, no protein drink, just three fossilized strawberries and a mason jar of flour.

The solution? Stock Mom's fridge and pantry with foods I actually eat. I realize after several trips back and forth to St. Louis that I'm surviving on three daily stops at the local convenience store, where nothing is healthy or sustainable. A quick grocery run makes all the difference. While perishables need replenishing each visit, at least I'll have a few staple items—soup, chips, and frozen breakfast bowls.

In the same way that keeping shampoo and laundry detergent stocked at Mom's is part of the strategy, having go-to foods with a long shelf life also brings a bit of normalcy to an otherwise chaotic situation.

BRINGING ALONG FUR FAMILY MEMBERS

Whether the trip is a flight from out of state or just a drive across town, personal routines are interrupted. My friend Chris experienced this too when she stayed with her mom. Because she needed to bring her pets, they had to work out a compromise in her mother's shed-free household. Here's her story.

Mom and Dad are divorced. They separated when I went away to college. Mom is very independent. She's in her seventies and still works full-time. I guess that's where I get my drive.

She'd been putting off hip replacement surgery for years, brushing it aside until the pain became impossible to ignore. It was affecting her quality of life. She stopped playing pickleball, wasn't driving much and was struggling to keep up with weekly chores like grocery shopping.

The doctor warned her: without surgery, she risked permanent damage and might have to give up the things she loved for good. That finally tipped the scales. She scheduled the procedure.

And she did great. In and out of the hospital quickly, breezed through rehab, and was back home before we knew it. Still, she wasn't quite ready to be on her own. I didn't feel comfortable leaving her until she was fully back on her feet, so I moved in for about a month.

Because my husband travels for work, I had to bring our dogs with me, Charlie the shepherd and Roxy the lab. Mom loves dogs, but she's never been a fan of shedding. She needed help and I needed to care for my dogs, so she compromised and welcomed Charlie and Roxy into her home.

The real challenge was her two-story condo and tiny backyard. Not exactly ideal for two big dogs with energy to burn. At home, I walk them regularly, but now I was walking them twice a day just to keep them settled. Honestly, the extra exercise was good for all of us.

Packing for the stay meant prepping a to-go bag for the dogs, too—bowls, beds, crates, food, leashes. It was a full operation. But settling in together, even with the chaos, felt like the right kind of disruption. We made it work.

Getting Stuff Done: Creating a Remote Office That Works

To balance my professional work responsibilities with my *mom* responsibilities, having a place to work at Mom's house is crucial. Unlike Mom, I relish the quiet. I'm most productive with silence, no TV, no music, just my thoughts and my computer.

Mom, on the other hand, has an incessant need to talk, even when I don't respond. I remember coming home from college on weekends and trying to study. It was impossible. Mom hated the silence. Being in the presence of others and not talking was unimaginable, maybe even impolite, in her mind.

To create my own private oasis, I set up my office in a spare bedroom, outfitting it with a folding table and chair that can be easily collapsed and stored under a bed, respecting her home when I'm not here.

With my *office furniture* in place, I make a trip to the local electronics store and purchase a full-size monitor, docking station, laptop stand, mouse pad, surge protector, network cables—the works — to configure my new space. I never thought a temporary workspace would bring me peace, but with uncertainty around me, this is just the getaway I need.

Setting Boundaries: Sharing Space and Honoring Our Differences

Along with easing travel hassles, having my own space and personal items at Mom's also requires setting healthy boundaries. I am her daughter, but I'm no longer a dependent child. I have an independent life with a husband, two grown sons, and a dog. And fighting to sustain my healthier life habits when I'm living in her home is challenging.

Frequent trips blur the lines of healthy living, and I quickly slip back into familiar patterns from my dysfunctional upbringing, such as being the family peacemaker between Tina and Mom or taking on the role of the adult when Mom refuses to make difficult decisions. Setting boundaries, like not eating Mom's food or using her laundry detergent, helps me cling to the sense of normalcy that anchors me to the life I've built in Texas. One with less conflict, more respect, and fewer alcohol-related behaviors. While compulsive traits still linger in my immediate family, we work every day to mitigate the unhealthy patterns inherited from our parents. We resolve conflicts diplomatically. We don't scream at each other. We say please and thank you and ask each other for help with kindness and tact. Our philosophy is that if we are going to be polite to a checker at the grocery store, we at least owe the same respect to those we love.

Compromise—We Are Both Breathing the Same Air

Fortunately for me, Mom gave up her two-pack-a-day habit when the first grandkid arrived, and she and Dad moved into a new house. Once she makes up her mind, her determination is unstoppable. No patch, no gum—she just quit. Cold turkey.

This isn't the case for Ruth. Her father is a chain smoker, and she needs to set boundaries for herself during her visits. Here's how she tells her story.

> Dad's been smoking since he was fifteen. He's tried quitting more times than I can count, but it's a hard thing to shake. He still loves the smell, the taste, the ritual of it. He's tried everything from nicotine gum, step-down patches; even gave hypnotherapy a shot once—but nothing stuck. He knows all the side effects, knows what it's doing to him, but it's his life and he's made peace with it.
>
> He's about an hour away, still in the same little farm town where I grew up. Mom's gone now, but he's holding steady in that same two-bedroom house. Health-wise, he's not doing too bad. Slowing down some, but he manages.

He always perks up when I come to visit. I usually stay for a week, help out where I can. The toilet doesn't get scrubbed unless I'm there, and I'll cook dinner a few nights. I always make Mom's cherry pie—her recipe, crust and all.

We've got an understanding, too. In exchange for me visiting, cooking and cleaning for him, he agrees to smoke outside. I've got a touch of COPD from growing up around secondhand smoke, and I just don't want it hanging in the air, especially cooped up in a small place like that. It's hard enough to breathe some days without adding smoke to the mix.

He doesn't fuss. He just steps out to the porch when he wants to light up.

No matter the setup—whether I'm staying with Mom for a long period of time or rotating in one week each month—I've learned that structure is everything. Setting boundaries, carving out a workspace and creating an environment where I can sleep well and eat decently makes the whole arrangement manageable.

Mom gets the support she needs. I stay present and accountable as part of her care team. And I hold onto a thread of familiarity from my 'other life' where I'm a wife, a mother and a full-time employee. It's not perfect, but it's a compromise that works—for both of us.

CHAPTER 9

Aging in Place—There's No Place Like Home

Topics

— **Aging in Place: What it Really Means**

— **Hiring In-Home Help: What Caregivers Do and What They Don't**

— **Aging in Place Hacks: Solutions that Make a Big Difference**

— **In-Home Rehab: Top 5 Safety Accommodations**

Many aging adults prefer to continue living in their own homes as they grow older, rather than transitioning to senior housing, such as an independent living or assisted living facility. This choice allows them to maintain their independence in an environment they find comfortable and meaningful. For some, their home is the last connection to a deceased spouse or the space where they raised their children, making it deeply sentimental.

While aging in place may be the dream scenario for the aging parent, it can be a tremendous burden for the aging parent's "project care team" because managing someone else's household and ensuring their needs are met is a full-time job, often involving the coordination of services, caregivers, and medical visits.

Aging in Place: What it Really Means

Aging in place can feel like Kansas for Dorothy in *The Wizard of Oz*. There is nothing as comforting as familiar surroundings and routines; truly, "There's no place like home." but for those managing their own households and coordinating aging parent care, this option can be unbearably stressful and exhausting.

For a time, aging in place may work well, especially for older adults in good health, those who are resourceful and self-sufficient, or individuals living with a supportive companion like a spouse or roommate. But even the most independent aging parent will eventually face moments when additional support becomes essential.

Whether it's recovering from knee surgery or regaining strength after a hospital stay for pneumonia, temporary setbacks can quickly shift daily routines. Tasks like getting to the bathroom safely or preparing a simple meal may require short- or long-term in-home assistance.

WHAT DOES THE PHRASE 'AGING IN PLACE' MEAN?

When I was 'hired' as the project manager of Mom's life, the phrase aging in place was unfamiliar. It simply means that an older adult chooses to stay in their own home as they age, rather than relocating to a facility or moving in with family.

For my mom, aging in place isn't just a preference— it is non-negotiable. She wants to stay rooted in the house she knows, surrounded by familiar walls and neighbors who wave from across the street. It's the place where she feels most herself.

Dad died several years ago, and Mom never truly grieved his loss. Her deep codependence keeps her tethered to the past, and the house they shared is her last tangible connection to him. Before his passing–and relentlessly since—Mom metaphorically 'clicks her heels together' and mumbles, 'There's no place like home. There's no place like home.' Her desire to remain in her home is, in her mind, the only option.

Since Dad's passing, my sister and I have committed to helping Mom hold onto her dream for as long as possible but living alone now without support is no longer sustainable. Changes are necessary to balance her desire for independence with our need for safety and care. One of our greatest concerns is her physical safety, particularly the risk of more frequent falls, a common and serious issue among aging adults.

> Falling incidents often stem from a combination of factors such as muscle loss, balance issues, low blood pressure, and conditions like osteoporosis. Osteoporosis, characterized by weak and brittle bones, becomes increasingly prevalent with age, especially among women after menopause. Lifestyle choices such as smoking, inactivity, poor nutrition, and excessive alcohol consumption can further inhibit bone formation and heighten the risk of falling.

Spanning several years, Mom has been in and out of the hospital as the result of two fall-related hip-replacement surgeries and occasional out-of-whack blood work. After each instance, she rehabs, sometimes followed by a stint in respite care, and sometimes by Medicare-provided nursing and physical therapy services in her home. Her latest fall notches things up to a whole new level.

This time, Mom's fall doesn't result in a broken arm or a dislocated knee. No, this time it is far worse. While attending a wedding shower, she missed a step leading into a sunken living room and fell. The impact fractured her C3 and C4 vertebrae. In simple terms, she broke her neck.

We consult two specialists, and both tell us that surgery isn't a practical option. Her age and the uncertain outcome make the risk too great. Her prognosis is delivered with clinical simplicity: proceed with caution, wear a neck brace, and live your life.

At first, this plan sounds manageable. But as days, weeks, and years pass, we begin to understand the magnitude of the prognosis. Beneath the seemingly straightforward treatment lies a slow, creeping reality, paralyzing neuropathy. The condition doesn't just limit movement; it reshapes daily life in ways we can't even imagine. She begins losing sensation in her hands, describing them as feeling "slick as glass." Her grip weakens. She drops things without even realizing it, like her daily medications, which end up scattered on the floor instead of making it to her mouth. Ordinary tasks grow risky. Pouring a cup of hot coffee, retrieving food from the microwave—these once-routine tasks now carry real danger.

The truth is that Mom needs help. Living alone without assistance is no longer safe. She's also not keeping up with personal hygiene. She skips meals. And still, she insists on staying in her home.

So, we find a middle ground: we bring in a caregiver. It's not the solution she imagined, but it's the one that allows her to stay where she feels most herself while giving her the support she now needs.

Convincing Mom—Caregivers Are a Must

Every situation is different and knowing when to bring in a caregiver for a parent who wants to age in place isn't always obvious. It often begins with small clues—expired milk in the fridge, a growing stack of unopened mail on the kitchen table. These quiet signals build over time, and eventually, the need for extra support becomes harder to ignore.

In our case, Mom's worsening neuropathy is just one piece of the puzzle. Her refrigerator is nearly bare. No fresh produce. No signs of balanced, protein-rich meals. When we look closer, we realize her diet has narrowed to coffee, oatmeal, beer, and pretzels, her personal version of the four essential food groups.

We begin to see other signs, too. With each passing week, Mom accumulates less laundry. There are no bath towels, no underwear, and we notice she often wears the same clothes for days on end. Her personal hygiene is clearly slipping. Something must change.

Our first hurdle is getting her to agree to a caregiver. Trust doesn't come easily. Despite her friendly, chatty demeanor, she's always on guard. Sometimes it's fear, worrying that someone might be scoping out her home for a future robbery. Other times, it's discomfort with the idea of accepting help, especially in relation to her personal care. Her caution is constant, and her reluctance to spend money on services she doesn't deem "essential" only adds to the challenge.

After countless conversations, careful negotiation, and more than a little pleading, we finally draw the line. We ultimately insist, "Mom, you must have regular, consistent caregiver support for your safety, for our peace of mind, and so you can age in place the way you want."

Hiring In-Home Help: What Caregivers Do and What They Don't

When it comes to hiring caregivers, two main paths typically emerge. One option is to work with an independent caregiver, someone who's branched out on their own after gaining experience with an agency, or who comes highly recommended through word of mouth as someone who genuinely enjoys supporting older adults. The other route involves partnering with a caregiving agency, a company that specializes in matching trained professionals with seniors who need assistance.

Each option has its own advantages and disadvantages, and throughout our journey caring for Mom, we've used both approaches at different times. Ultimately, the right choice depends on individual needs, the senior's preferences and health requirements.

Our first experience hiring a caregiving company is a wake-up call. Like most parts of my role as "project manager of Mom's life," I'm figuring things out as I go. One thing becomes clear almost immediately: the polished website images of radiant caregivers and cheerful elders don't reflect our reality. Adjusting expectations is essential because the gap between marketing and lived experience is wide.

Our initial point of contact is the company's social worker, who describes the caregiver matching process as something akin to speed dating. She meets with Mom, learns her preferences and personality, and finds her ideal match. "Like speed dating," she says, "It might take a few tries." But she reassures us that Mom's caregiving "soulmate" is out there.

It all sounds fantastic, and I'm eager to dive in. Sign me up. How can I help? Knowing Mom's likes and dislikes, I'm confident we can streamline the process. All we need are caregiver bios or résumés. With experience hiring contractors and staff in our professional lives, my sister and I are well-equipped to assist. We can even pre-interview candidates, making sure only the strongest contenders get introduced to Mom, which can weed out poor matches and limit her opportunity to veto every single candidate, especially since she's not exactly thrilled about the idea to begin with.

It feels like a solid, collaborative plan. But wow, am I naïve. I quickly learn there's no roster of caregivers "waiting in the wings." This company operates more like a contracting service, recruiting new caregivers only after they've signed on a new client.

Eventually, we give in to the "speed dating" model. Over the next several weeks, the social worker lines up a series of "probable suitors" for Mom. Each time, she dismisses them. *She lacks compassion. She isn't genuine. She acts like I'm a bother. She's as old as I am.*

To be fair, Mom isn't wrong.

From what we see, the caregiver candidate pool tends to fall into two camps. On one end are first or second semester CNA (certified nursing assistant) students with minimal life experiences and little in common with our 83-year-old mother. On the other end are retirees, former nurses about Mom's age, looking to stay active and give back.

Finally, a "reasonable" match surfaces, and Mom clicks with Nicole. She agrees to a second visit, a small but meaningful win. Determined to get her money's worth, Mom drafts a to-do list of chores for Nicole to tackle. This isn't exactly the caregiving arrangement we imagined, but whatever it takes to get Mom's buy-in, we'll take it.

Nicole returns and her 'tragic flaw' is unveiled; she doesn't know how to iron. Top of Mom's chore list—press sheer kitchen curtains. She lights up at the chance to teach Nicole the art of perfect ironing. I can only imagine the level of detail, just as we were taught growing up: *take your time, never let the curtain touch the floor, align the edges perfectly.*

Despite Mom's masterclass in textile care, Nicole's debut ends in disaster. She leaves the iron in place too long, burning a hole straight through the center of the beloved curtains.

Mom's verdict? "We aren't compatible."

And just like that, the search resumes. *Swipe right.*

BACK TO THE CAREGIVER CANDIDATE POOL

With Nicole out of the picture, a new round of 'eligible' caregivers cycle through. A few earn second or even third visits, but none make the cut. Take CeCe, for example, a caregiver Mom genuinely tries to make work. Thanks to the in-home camera system, we get a front-row seat to Cece's version of completing 'light housekeeping' chores. Who knew you could dust bedroom furniture by standing in the middle of the room, scrolling your phone, and lazily waving a feather duster in the general direction of a nightstand?

Then came Allison, who dropped her bag on the counter, wandered into Mom's den, and without a word, curled up on the couch for a nap.

In the months that followed, we cycled through caregivers who were, at best, adequate. Not ideal, but passable. Just as we begin settling in with someone who seems to fit, they quit, realizing: "This isn't the job I thought it would be."

Our experience with hiring in-home caregivers isn't unique. My friend, Carla, shared a similar story.

> Agency placements can be iffy arrangements. We once had a lovely young woman who bonded with Grandma and was generally a great fit, but she had a troubled son, and as a single mom, would often go absent without notice.
>
> This left me in a pinch with no emergency substitute on more than one occasion. I had to drop whatever I had planned to be present for that day or stretch of days. I ultimately quit my part-time job, because I couldn't depend on our caregiver.
>
> Eventually, we found a much more reliable, quality person to care for Grandma. We found her independently, rather than through an agency. She had years of experience and loved the work she did. She had a gift for caring for aging adults and stayed with us for several years.

Mom's Perfect Match

We went through caregiver after caregiver, each one falling short until we met the one—Sandy. From the moment she stepped into Mom's world, something shifted. Sandy wasn't just capable; she was kind, articulate, and profoundly respectful. It was as if the two of them had known each other their whole lives.

They clicked instantly. A quiet admiration passed between them, growing into a bond that felt more like friendship than duty. Sandy listened with genuine interest as Mom shared her hard-earned lessons on raising children, managing a household, and navigating life with grace. And Mom, in turn, lit up with purpose, delighted to pass along what she knew. Sandy wasn't just a good fit. She was the right one—the kind of caregiver we all hope for but seldom find.

Mom and Sandy quickly became inseparable. Mom's meticulous habits—stacking plastic containers with geometric precision or declaring that vacuuming only counts if the carpet lines run perfectly parallel—might have rattled a lesser soul. But Sandy met every quirk with quiet grace. She didn't just tolerate Mom's routines; she respected them.

In return, Mom recognized Sandy's patience and unwavering care. What began as a working relationship blossomed into something deeper. They filled a space in each other's lives that neither had known was empty, forming a bond that was both tender and quietly profound. Watching them together was like witnessing something rare and deeply right.

When hiring private caregivers, it's important to consider how their earnings will be reported for tax purposes. Will the caregiver be classified as a 1099 contractor or as a household employee? This distinction affects both tax reporting and the overall cost of care.

MOM'S SECRET KEEPER

Mom and Sandy's relationship felt less like caregiver and client, and more like two middle school best friends, laughing and confiding in each other. Inseparable. It was perfect until it wasn't.

Trust, as wonderful as it is, can sometimes cloud judgment, and that's exactly what happened with Sandy. One afternoon, she arrived for her shift and immediately sensed something was off. Mom was using her walker, a device she hadn't touched in months, since regaining full mobility after her hip replacement. Concerned, Sandy gently asked what had happened. It took some coaxing, but eventually, the truth came out: Mom had fallen while pushing her cart in the grocery store parking lot.

Panicked and embarrassed, Mom begged Sandy not to tell me or my sister. Sandy, torn between loyalty and responsibility, finally agreed, on one condition: Mom had to have an X-ray.

But fate intervened. Sandy's daughter fell ill at school, and Sandy had to leave early. Mom insisted she'd be fine, assuring Sandy that she'd already been walking like this for a week. The fall had happened the previous Wednesday.

Still conflicted, Sandy made a promise: she'd keep the secret for one night. But when she returned the next day, they would tell us together. That was the deal.

After that incident, our gratitude for their bond was tempered by concern. Sandy's closeness with Mom had blurred the boundaries of her role. In choosing to keep Mom's secret, she let personal loyalty override clinical judgment.

She stayed on for several more months, continuing to care for Mom with the same warmth and attentiveness. But, for us, the dynamic had shifted. We found ourselves watching more closely, no longer fully confident in her professional distance. Eventually, Sandy left for a better-paying job outside the caregiving field. In the meantime, we adopted a quiet policy: trust but verify.

ASKING THE RIGHT QUESTIONS

One of the most important lessons we've learned along the way is this: whether hiring an independent caregiver or partnering with a professional agency, asking the right questions matters. Thoughtful, informed conversations can make all the difference.

> **Top Questions to Ask When Hiring a Caregiver.**
>
> 1. Are caregivers bonded and background-checked?
>
> 2. What services do caregivers provide—and what are they not allowed to do?
>
> 3. If the client needs help to be lifted or transferred, is the caregiver trained to assist?
>
> 4. What certifications or formal training do caregivers have?

5. Does the company offer its own caregiver training? If so, what does it include?

6. How are caregivers supervised or monitored on the job?

7. For medical needs and daily living activities, what specific tasks will the caregiver handle?

8. Can caregivers organize medications by day or week? Are they trained to check vital signs like blood pressure?

9. Are caregivers able to schedule and coordinate appointments, such as doctor visits or physical therapy?

10. Can caregivers shop for groceries or pick up supplies? If so, how are purchases handled—do we provide a gift card or reimbursement?

11. Is there an extra charge for mileage or gas when caregivers run errands or travel to appointments?

12. Can caregivers accompany the client to medical appointments? If the appointment runs long, will they stay until the client returns home?

13. What's the minimum shift length a caregiver will work?

14. What's the maximum number of hours a caregiver can work in one shift?

15. If a caregiver is unavailable, will a backup be provided?

16. How much notice is given if a substitute caregiver will be filling in?

17. Are in-home cameras permitted, and if so, are there any restrictions?

18. What counts as "light housekeeping," and which tasks will the caregiver actually perform?

19. If the client falls while under the caregiver's supervision, what steps are taken?

20. How are services billed, and what forms of payment are accepted?

21. What's the policy on client cancellations?

22. Are caregivers allowed to drive the client's car?

23. Can the client ride in the caregiver's car?

24. What happens if there's a car accident while transporting the client?

25. If the client has concerns about the caregiver's performance, what's the process for addressing them?

Aging in Place Hacks

Hiring in-home caregivers is just one piece of the puzzle when supporting a parent's desire to age in place. A wide range of resources can help make this goal more achievable, including emergency alert systems, pre-portioned meal services, and in-home delivery options are just a few tools that add safety and convenience.

A Bird's Eye View

Even with a daily caregiver schedule in place, there are still stretches of time when Mom is alone. While she doesn't need around-the-clock care and remains largely self-sufficient, that doesn't ease our concern.

To better ensure her safety, we install cameras throughout the house, three in the kitchen, one in the bedroom, and several positioned to cover key hallways. For me, living out of state, these cameras are a lifeline. When I can't reach her or just need peace of mind, I open the app and check in. We've kept the microphones off to preserve her privacy during caregiver visits, but the two-way audio feature allows us to speak to her if needed.

While this monitoring provides reassurance, it has its drawbacks, especially when my OCD tendencies kick in. Some mornings, before my feet even touch the floor, I instinctively check Mom's cameras to confirm all is well.

One morning, as I tune in, I see Mom steadying herself as she gets out of bed. She moves around the end of the bed, and suddenly, almost in slow motion, I watch her fall forward, disappearing from the camera's view. Frozen, I remain glued to the small screen until she eventually pulls herself up, settling into a seated position on the bed. Once I'm sure she's okay, I immediately call her cordless phone, knowing it's always within arm's reach on her bed each night.

Moments like these remind me that once you take on the role of caregiver for an aging parent, you're always on call, constantly on high alert and worrying.

MEDICAL ALERT SYSTEM MISHAP

Along with the in-home camera system, we insist Mom wear a medical alert device, a simple pendant designed to summon help in case of a fall or health emergency. Many models offer features like automatic fall detection, GPS tracking, and two-way communication.

But as with any technology, glitches happen. During setup, Mom worked with the dispatcher to test the system. It didn't take long to discover just how sensitive the device was. Within days, she received a call from local first responders. An alert had been triggered at the firehouse. Mortified, Mom apologized and vowed to keep the pendant nearby but not actually wear it.

I remind her that leaving it 'sitting on the kitchen table' serves no purpose and won't help anyone in an emergency. Reluctantly, she agrees to keep it with her. However, after hearing the nerve-racking account of her latest ordeal, I finally concede and support her decision to end the contract and return the device.

Here is how her story unfolded.

> I was getting ready to take a shower and placed the medical necklace carefully on the bathroom counter, right next to the towel, making sure not to jostle it. As I rinsed shampoo from my hair, the bathroom door suddenly flew open. I nearly collapsed from the shock. I was the only one at home. And then, out of nowhere, I heard a man's voice. I opened my eyes, suds streaming down my face, and there he was, a tall, muscular firefighter standing in my bathroom.
>
> I was horrified and yelled at him to get out. He explained that they'd been dispatched for a medical emergency and, when no one answered the phone, they came to check if I was okay. I told him I was fine, just scared and embarrassed.
>
> "That's it," Mom said resolutely. "I'm done. I'm not using that thing anymore. Enough is enough. I'm sending it back."

While ensuring your aging parent's safety is crucial, flexibility and compromise are often necessary. For your parent to respect and value your guidance, you must also be understanding when something feels unreasonable to them. In our case, the medical alert system wasn't functioning properly, and Mom's dignity and pride were at stake.

In-Home Rehab: Top 5 Safety Accommodations

PT, OT AND NURSING SUPPORT FOLLOWING A HOSPITAL STAY

After multiple hospitalizations, rehab stays, and homecomings with Mom, we learned an important lesson: Medicare often includes in-home evaluations and follow-up support for those recovering at home.

A nurse or evaluation team typically visits the home to assess safety and recommend changes like removing throw rugs that might slip, rearranging furniture, or clearing pathways to reduce fall risks. If needed, physical and occupational therapists can be scheduled to provide rehabilitation right in the home.

Nursing services may also be available to assist with medication management, monitor blood pressure or glucose levels, and offer other clinical support.

These services are invaluable in promoting recovery and independence. Still, it's important to remember they don't replace the broader role of a caregiver. Tasks like bathing, meal prep, and transportation to appointments may still require additional help.

Top 5 Safety In-Home Accommodations

- Eliminate Step Stools and Keep Essentials Within Reach

  Store frequently used items (dishes, medications, clothing) at waist-to-shoulder height

  Avoid high shelves or low cabinets that require bending or climbing

- Install Grab Bars in Key Areas

  Place sturdy grab bars in bathrooms
  (near toilets, showers, and tubs)

  Ensure they're professionally anchored, not suction-based, for reliable support

- Secure Railings at All Entry/Exit Points

  Add railings on both sides of stairs and steps, including garage and porch entries

  Extend railings beyond the first and last step
  for added stability

- Improve Lighting & Remove Hazards

  Have bright, glare-free lighting in hallways, stairwells, and entryways

  Add nightlights in bedrooms and bathrooms

  Remove loose rugs, cords, or clutter that
  can cause tripping

- Create a Slip-Resistant Environment

  Use non-slip mats in bathrooms and kitchens

  Ensure shoes and slippers have good traction

OPTIMIZING DELIVERY SERVICE

Beyond smart tech and caregiver support, home delivery services can play a vital role in helping aging adults stay safe and independent. If a parent is recovering from surgery or no longer driving, grocery delivery is a simple way to keep their kitchen stocked. Even if they're not tech-savvy, you can place the order for them. Services like store delivery options make it easy to send fresh produce, pantry staples, and nourishing meals straight to their door.

And don't forget to include her favorite treats. Whether it's cookies, ice cream, or that beloved hazelnut creamer, adding a few favorite treats can turn a routine delivery into a small act of joy. Sure, they might grumble about the delivery fees but resting easier knowing they're well-fed and safe at home is worth it.

Take a playbook page from your Gen Z family member and introduce your mom or dad to meal services. They will get nutritious, ready-to-eat meals, and you can rest easy knowing they are eating well.

Even if an aging parent still drives, bad weather can make errands risky. A quick grocery order can cover essentials like bread and milk without putting them in harm's way. My mom's guilty pleasure is Little Caesar's pizza, but she's reluctant to go out after dark. More than once, I've used DoorDash to send her a pepperoni pizza and breadsticks on a chilly Saturday night. It's always a hit. Another great option: pre-portioned, chef-prepared meal plans delivered right to her doorstep. These services offer fresh, balanced meals that are easy to heat and enjoy, no prep required.

Stay Curious—Seek Out Services

Supporting an aging parent often means thinking beyond the basics. There are specialized services available, especially for veterans, that can make a meaningful difference.

While searching for a way to donate durable medical equipment (DME), we came across a remarkable center that refurbishes and redistributes items like walkers and wheelchairs free of charge. Their mission is to support veterans, individuals experiencing homelessness, and others without access to essential mobility aids. The agency we found is located in St. Louis—check your local area for similar services.

Another practical tip: consider arranging laundry pickup and delivery. If your parent struggles to keep up with laundry because of mobility issues or a lack of energy, a local service can ease the burden while preserving their dignity.

> *There's a fine line between helping and over-helping. If a loved one is managing tasks, albeit slowly, but remains safe and feels self-sufficient, it may be best to let them do things their way. Independence, even in small doses, can be deeply empowering.*

It's Not a Hands-Off Experience

Helping your aging parent maintain their wish to age in place and stay in their home requires ongoing involvement, even with outside caregiving support in place. It's far from a hands-off arrangement. There's still a lot to manage and stay engaged with. While having a caregiver check in on a loved one a few times a week can be helpful, responsibilities like coordinating doctor visits, arranging or adjusting physical therapy schedules, and finding someone to repair the front porch light may still fall to you. Some caregivers may be able to assist with certain tasks, but it's important to adjust your expectations—this isn't a 'set it and forget it' solution.

CHAPTER 10

Making Tough Decisions When She Can't or Won't

Topics

— **Familiar Routines: The Chores They Loved and Why It's Time to Step In**

— **Driving Decisions: When Safety Outweighs Independence**

— **A Turning Point: Caregiving at 23**

— **Moving Parents In: Conversations and Considerations**

WHEN YOUR BEST EFFORTS AREN'T ENOUGH

When even your most diligent and exhaustive efforts fall short, it may be time to make tough decisions that Mom can't or won't. While some aging parents may find relief in being given 'permission' to let go of a big house filled with isolation and loneliness, this is not the case with our mom. Despite preparing and freezing carefully portioned meals, scheduling regular caregiver visits, and monitoring Mom's every move through cameras in her home, she still needs more help. Her refrigerator is empty. Canned goods in the pantry are three years past their expiration date. She rarely changes her clothes or bathes, and there is no telling the last time the toilet or shower was scrubbed. Our lives are out of whack. Our families are consumed with helping Mom live out her best elder years, and it is killing us.

Six lives have been upended—my sister's, my nephew's, my husband's, my two sons' and mine—all to accommodate my mom's desire to remain in her home. Tina and I work tirelessly to support her wish to age in place for as long as possible, but when your best 200 percent efforts are no longer enough, it may be time to make tough decisions that she can't or won't make. We've subtly and not so subtly broached the subject of Mom aging and the importance of making plans for her future somewhere other than her three-thousand square foot home, but she's not budging. And the more involved we become in her life, the more often we argue.

We first 'infiltrate' Mom's life by managing her household finances, with Tina handling the monthly bills. Although Mom's mind remains sharp and she enjoys tasks like balancing her checkbook, overdue credit card bills and unpaid HOA fees force an intervention. Additionally, we know that paying for caregivers and regular pest control treatments frustrates her, and left to her own devices, she would refuse to pay for these services. But, in the end, despite her resistance to change, Mom knows deep down that she needs help, even if she struggles to admit it.

Familiar Routines: The Chores They Loved and Why It's Time to Step In

Time, distance and reflection award us perspective, but in the heat of the moment, when Mom digs in her heels and refuses help, there is a lot of, as we say in business, *cussin' and discussin'* going on. Mom is stubborn and resistant. When we suggest and ultimately mandate that she hire someone to mow her yard, seasonally treat her lawn, and trim her bushes, you would think we were sending her to the gallows.

"I can spray for spiders," she argues. "And I can spread weed killer myself," she protests. "They sell weed and seed at Aldi."

She fights us every step of the way. Her mental fortitude is *her* blessing and *our* curse. Admirable? Yes. Unrealistic? Yes. A woman who struggles with balance issues and is prone to falling has no business mowing her lawn, no matter how small it is, yet she fails to see the problem.

Despite leveraging every change management technique we know—psychology, engagement, empowerment, logic—we even throw in some good old-fashion Catholic guilt—nothing works. Mom resists. She denies that she can't keep up with things she's always done and *if you don't talk about it or think about it, it won't happen.*

After relentless negotiations and cajoling, I lay down the law. "You are no longer cutting your own lawn because I said so. You will pay someone to do it. You can research the service, but it needs to be a professional lawn service and not the twelve-year-old who might have a baseball game that conflicts with mowing day. We need a consistent, reliable service."

This isn't the first nor the last conversation we'll have over lawn service. Mom's stubbornness undermines every lawn crew we bring in, even the ones she picks herself. No one is ever good enough. She criticizes them for not bagging the grass or blowing the clippings into the yard instead of sweeping them up. One time she cancels the professional service altogether, replacing them with t*he boy up the street who needs money for the summer.* Maddening.

REFLECTION—STRIVE TO SEE PAST THE PRESENT—WHAT IS IT MOM REALLY SAYING?

Growing up, Mom and Dad spent countless hours mowing, trimming, and perfecting the small lawn of their starter home, where we lived as a family until my sister and I went to college. While they both took pride in their home, Mom was especially passionate about the lawn. She strived for a perfectly manicured yard, one that resembled a golf course. And the landscaped flower beds needed to be equally flawless. One summer, she painted large decorative rocks white to complement the house—a move the neighbors never let her forget.

Eventually, my parents upgraded to their dream home in a high-end neighborhood with an HOA, where rows of pristine lawns resembled the country club fairways. Mom loved how beautiful her neighborhood looked, but her fierce competitive spirit drove her to outdo everyone, striving for the most impeccable yard on the block.

When we insist she can no longer care for the lawn, it breaks her heart. Only years later do I grasp what I'm asking her to surrender. The heavy mower, the uneven ground, the upkeep of equipment—all of it had become too demanding. Yet her longing to see the lawn she loves kept in perfect condition remains.

The challenge is that Mom finds joy in the journey. For her, the fun is the work. She loves being outdoors, tending to her lawn and pulling weeds from the sidewalk cracks. Being one with nature is her happy place. It brings her peace, and by removing this chore, we are unintentionally taking a part of her soul. Though she can't fully explain this, her resistance and defiance speak volumes. At a deeper level, every attempt to help her feels like we are chipping away at what made her, her.

When you are at your limit—exhausted, angry, frustrated and overwhelmed with this role you never signed up for and never wanted—try to pause and create some space. Conversations in the heat of the moment might not serve you or your aging parent well. Instead, focus on understanding the underlying message behind their words or actions. While you still may need to make tough decisions and implement plans they may resist, recognizing the motivation behind a loved one's behavior can bring clarity and reassurance for both of you.

Driving Decisions: When Safety Outweighs Independence

Driving is another contentious topic when it comes to supporting aging parents. Mom insists, "I know my body. I know when I can't drive anymore, and I'll be the first to admit it." While I'd like to believe that, her persistence for independence brings sound judgment and decision making into question.

The bittersweet of Mom's chronic osteoporosis and neuropathy spares us from having the difficult "we need to take your keys away" conversation. The situation resolves itself naturally, and we avoid the 'battle of wills' over the keys.

That's not the case for many others. It wasn't the case with our grandmother, nor with a friend of mine navigating a similar challenge while caring for her aging father.

When my grandmother was in independent living and her dementia progressed into Alzheimer's nearly overnight, my parents received a call from the local police department. She had driven to a convenience store to buy cigarettes for her husband, only to forget how to get home. Her husband had passed away years earlier, and her midnight excursion resulted in the police being called to the store two blocks from her apartment.

After safely getting my grandmother home, my dad made the decision to take her car keys. She never drove again, despite her protests and accusations that my father had stolen her car. She was no longer safe behind the wheel—for her own well-being and for the safety of others.

Stories such as these are all too common. A friend, Kim, is caring for her aging father, a fiercely determined man. Here is her story when her father resisted surrendering the car keys.

One morning, Kim's dad decided to visit his brother and set off on a cross-country trip from Texas to Illinois. He never made it to Illinois. Somewhere in the middle of Missouri, he took a wrong turn and ended up in Iowa. With his bank account nearly drained, he turned around and headed back toward Texas, only to miss another exit and wind-up 800 miles farther west than he intended. Out of gas and with a dead cell phone, he found himself stranded roadside.

Thankfully, a good Samaritan came to his aid, helped charge his phone, and contacted Kim. Grateful for the stranger's kindness, Kim sent funds electronically to refuel her father's car, and she asked the kind stranger to turn him around and point him east.

With his phone fully charged, Kim could once again track his movements. As he neared the correct turn off, Kim and her husband were standing roadside waving him down— pointing at the exit for him to turn right. Fortunately, he made it home safely.

Despite the ordeal, Kim's dad refused to surrender his car keys. Since he is a veteran, she sought the help of the local Veteran's Administration (VA) services which required that he successfully complete a series of driving tests, including a

> two-mile round trip from his apartment to a pancake house
> and back with an instructor riding along. When he couldn't
> determine if he needed to turn left or right out of the parking
> lot, he knew his time behind the wheel was over. It was a
> heartbreaking moment. Driving had been a cherished part
> of his independence, and he struggled, like so many aging
> adults, to relinquish the freedom and adjust to a life with
> restrictions and fewer options.

Addressing sensitive issues, like the decision to stop driving, is far less contentious when discussed early. Before reaching the point of "taking away the keys," have a conversation with your aging parent. Talk about the risks older adults may pose when driving becomes unsafe—whether due to slowed reaction times, impaired judgment, vision loss, or forgetfulness. Explore alternative transportation options, such as local bus services or ride-sharing programs, to help them maintain mobility and stay active.

A Turning Point: Caregiving at 23

The weight of helping Mom age in place hits me one Saturday evening when I check in on her via the home monitoring cameras. On this particular Saturday night, the caregiver called in sick, so my twenty-three-year-old nephew, stepped in for 'grandma duty.'

I watch him carefully place the cordless phone in the center of the bed. He leaves the room and returns with a cup of water. I watch as he secures the lid and bends the straw just right. He kisses her on the forehead before leaving the room. His genuine care is touching, but it hurts my soul.

This isn't a twenty-three-year-old's responsibility. He should be spending time with friends, gaming, or even relaxing at home watching a movie, not tending to his aging grandmother. Loving her and playing dominoes on a Saturday afternoon is one thing, but being her nursemaid and putting her to bed shouldn't fall to him.

Mom's insistence on staying in her home is pushing all of us to do more than we can handle. What Tina and I are asking of our families is unfair. And Mom's aging in place 'solution' is stretching all of us to our limits. *Doesn't she see the toll it is taking on all of us? How can she be so self-centered?*

My nephew's Saturday night caregiver shift is a breaking point for me. Things must change. My next scheduled trip is a week away. Mom and I need to have an honest conversation.

THE TALK

The following weekend, I arrive in town and spend much of Saturday grocery shopping, cooking and portioning healthy meals that Mom or her caregivers can pull out of the freezer and heat up.

For dinner that night, I prepare pasta and salad–a big mistake. Mom's neuropathy makes it nearly impossible for her to hold a fork steady, let alone keep slippery spaghetti from sliding off her plate. Yet, she is determined to feed herself, and she's grateful for the meal I've prepared.

After cleaning the floor around her chair and wiping bits of dinner from her shirt, I launch into *the talk*.

We start with pleasantries—Mom thanking me for visiting so often and acknowledging how difficult it must be for Rick and the boys. I agree. *Yes, this is very difficult for all of us.* Mom tries to assure me I don't need to worry about her. She can take care of herself.

I push back. "No, Mom, you can't." I tell her. "You need help. You have caregivers, and we're all doing everything we can to support you, but it's just too much. Something's got to change."

Tears well up in her eyes. "I just wish I could help you and Tina. I don't want to be a burden."

Here is my opening.

"Do you really mean that?"

"Of course I do," she replies.

"Then we need to make a change. We need you to move. It's time to find an assisted-living facility."

"No!" she screams, her voice shaking with emotion. "I am not moving into one of those places! I hate them. I want to die here, in my home. This is where your father died…" She breaks into sobs.

"Mom," I say softly, "this isn't something I'm doing to you. We know how much it means to you to stay in your home for as long as possible, but it's becoming impossible. You said yourself; this is taking a toll on Tina and me."

"You can't make me move! I have rights!" she yells in anger.

This isn't how I want the evening to end. *How am I ever going to get her out of this house?*

I have finally addressed the topic we've been avoiding for years; Mom needs to move. I hate her reaction, and yet I feel somehow liberated. True to my role as the eternal peacemaker, I steer the conversation to safer ground, restore a sense of calm, and help her get ready for bed. For now, nothing changes, but the subject has been raised.

To help with family communication, guidance with living accommodations and difficult conversations with aging parents, consider recruiting the support of a concierge senior living advisor, sometimes known as a Certified Senior Care & Transition Advisor.

This advisor is a paid professional who provides personalized guidance to older adults and their families in choosing the right senior living option, such as independent living, assisted living, memory care, or skilled nursing, based on health needs, lifestyle preferences, and budget.

What They Do

- Personalized Assessments: Advisors meet with seniors and families to understand medical conditions, daily living needs, emotional preferences, and financial constraints.

- Tailored Recommendations: They curate a shortlist of senior living communities or care options that align with the individual's requirements.

- Navigation Support: Because the senior living landscape can be overwhelming, advisors simplify the process, explain differences between care levels, and help families avoid costly mistakes.

- Transition Assistance: They often coordinate tours, assist with paperwork, and provide ongoing support during the move.

- Advocacy & Resources: Many advisors also connect families with additional services such as in-home care, financial aid programs, or veteran benefits.

WHY FAMILIES USE THEM

- Expertise: They know the local senior living communities and can quickly identify safe, reputable options.

- Stress Reduction: Families avoid the burden of researching dozens of facilities on their own.

- Peace of Mind: Seniors and caregivers gain confidence that decisions are informed and compassionate.

- Cost Awareness: Advisors help families understand pricing structures and available financial assistance.

Moving Parents In: Conversations and Considerations

For some, living with an aging parent may be an option. Not for us. Having Mom move in with my sister, who lives nearby, isn't realistic. Tina has a two-story home with all the bedrooms upstairs, which is hardly ideal for an aging parent with mobility issues. Beyond logistics, the emotional strain is too much. Their relationship is already fragile, and adding the stress of daily caregiving could push it past the breaking point.

We've prepared our home with the thought that Mom might one day move in with us. But relocating to Texas ultimately isn't a viable option. Naturally anxious and deeply resistant to change, she relies on her doctors, friends and familiar surroundings to feel grounded. Uprooting her would strip away that stability and heighten her anxiety. Remaining in St. Louis is the best choice for Mom—leaving me to shoulder the growing challenges of monthly trips between Texas and Missouri, caregiving from a distance.

Living with aging parents should only be considered after honest self-assessment and open family discussions about the potential pros and cons, including financial implications, the impact on family dynamics, the level of care needed, and each person's desire for independence. While living together can strengthen relationships and provide valuable time together, it can also lead to increased stress. Therefore, it is crucial to evaluate whether a multi-generational home is a suitable and sustainable option for everyone involved.

Before deciding to live with an aging parent, consider these questions:

- Your Parent's Needs

  What is their current health status, including chronic conditions or cognitive decline?

  Can you provide the necessary care and manage their medical issues?

  Will they have adequate space and privacy for independence?

- Your Family's Situation

  How well do you and your parent get along, and can you resolve differences?

  How will cohabitation affect your own health, your marriage, and your children?

  Are you prepared for increased responsibilities, a potential loss of personal time, and the financial implications?

- The Practicalities

  Are your home modifications safe and manageable for an aging person?

  Can you have open and honest discussions about finances and caregiving responsibilities?

- The Parent's Perspective

  Are you prepared for potential challenges if your parent struggles to transition from being the head of their own household to a secondary role?

  Will they accept your assistance, or will they feel a loss of control and independence?

CONVERSATION STARTERS

Discussions about significant life changes, like taking away car keys or moving a parent into assisted living, can be uncomfortable, especially in strained relationships. It helps to address these topics before tough decisions become urgent. With my dad, conversations such as these were easier. He was more open, but not my mom. Starting with indirect examples, like discussing the situation of a friend or relative, can be less confrontational. Saying something like, "Can you believe Uncle Russ is still driving? His eyesight isn't what it used to be. Someone really should step in and take his keys," can gently introduce the subject and pave the way to discuss how your parent perceives their own aging journey.

Other important topics to approach include selling the family home, inheritance plans, and funeral preferences. These discussions should be gradual. Rarely can everything be resolved in a single conversation. For example, while walking with my dad after his surgery, I casually asked, "What are your thoughts? At one point, you mentioned not wanting to be buried." Without hesitation, he replied, "No, burial doesn't make sense to me. It costs too much, and it's not good for the earth. I think I'd like to be cremated and placed in the church's columbarium wall." And that was that—his wishes were clear and decided.

A few months after 'the talk,' Mom fell in her home with a caregiver present. It was a fluke accident but became the catalyst for her transition to an assisted-living facility after another stay in the hospital.

RESOURCES

Caregiving at Home: A Guide to Community Resources

CHAPTER 11

Senior Living Accommodations— What Differentiates One from Another?

Topics

— Senior Living 101: Understanding Assisted Living, Long-Term Care, and More

— Beyond the Basics: Comparing Services and Support Levels

— Planning for the Price Tag: Navigating Costs, Insurance and VA Benefits

Talking about senior living arrangements has always been taboo with Mom. She refuses to face the realities of aging or even consider downsizing and leaving her home. She has long imagined spending her remaining years there. "Your dad died here. I want to die here, too," she reminds me daily. But as her health declines, that hope becomes less and less realistic. Despite her reluctance, my sister and I still need to understand how one type of facility differs from another.

Similar to learning an entirely new vocabulary related to medical terms and geriatric lingo, I now must learn about senior living options. Understanding the nuances differentiating independent living and assisted living, untangling the often-interchangeable use of terms like skilled nursing, long-term care facilities, and nursing homes, understanding the terms of long-term care insurance, and grasping the costs associated with senior living accommodations send me down another rabbit hole and closer to another course credit in my degree as Project Manager of Mom.

SHE'S BEEN IN RESPITE CARE FOR THREE MONTHS— IS IT TIME TO MAKE THE BREAK?

Mom has somewhat adjusted to respite care, at least as much as we can hope for. She's still resistant and ornery, and despite the staff's optimism about how 'Most who come here acclimate after a while,' she remains steadfast in her desire to return home. The *only* part of the experience she genuinely enjoys is Lady, the black lab. Mom keeps a stash of dog bones in her room, ensuring Lady finds her way down the hall and settles in for the night on the floor beside her bed.

In the corporate world, I am frequently reminded that *hope is not a strategy*, but I'm 'hopeful' that Mom will open her mind and heart to the idea of making this senior living community her new, permanent home, whether in the independent living portion of the complex or in the assisted living section. It just makes sense. She's been away from her home for a few months now, following a hip replacement surgery, rehab and now respite care. She's regained her strength, and she can easily move into one of the apartments. From my perspective, it's ideal—small enough to support her independence, yet close enough to medical staff for peace of mind. And with other residents close by, she can make friends and engage in social activities to keep her mind sharp, helping to stave off loneliness and the risk of mental decline.

Senior Living 101: Understanding Assisted Living, Long-Term Care, and More

Similar to this beautiful facility where Mom is staying, senior living communities exist throughout the country. These communities provide residential housing designed specifically for older adults, typically those aged fifty-five and above. They offer a range of amenities, services, and activities tailored to seniors' needs and preferences, including independent living, assisted living, and other specialized care options. Designed to support health, well-being, and independence, these communities create environments where seniors can thrive. Let's explore the various senior living accommodations and how each differs in purpose and support.

INDEPENDENT LIVING

Independent living encompasses a range of all-inclusive housing options, commonly known as retirement communities, senior living communities, or continuing care retirement communities (CCRCs). These residences are designed for healthy older adults who can live independently while minimizing the responsibilities of home maintenance.

These communities vary in size and structure, offering residents the flexibility to choose between private apartments or detached homes, often with shared spaces that foster social engagement and convenience. Residents personalize their spaces with their own furniture, household items and personal belongings, creating a home with fewer responsibilities and a simpler lifestyle compared to traditional homeownership.

AMENITIES AND SERVICES

Independent living communities are designed to enhance quality of life while providing supportive services. Common amenities include:

- Dining options—Shared dining areas with optional prepared meals
- Recreation & social activities—On-site events, clubs, and entertainment
- Convenient services—Banking, beauty salons, and fitness centers
- Transportation—Shuttle services for errands and appointments
- Housekeeping & laundry—Light cleaning and linen services
- Safety & security—24-hour staff presence for added peace of mind

Many communities welcome residents' pets, provided they can still care for them. Studies show that pets provide emotional and social support, helping reduce loneliness among older adults. However, pet policies may vary based on the facility, so it's important to check for restrictions on breed, size, and the number of pets allowed.

Seniors may reside in an independent living facility for months or years, depending on their individual needs and ability to continue living safely on their own. Many residents still drive and some remain employed, with certain facilities offering designated, covered parking spaces.

Assisted Living

Assessing how assisted living facilities differ from independent living facilities, assisted living is a long-term care option for individuals who typically need help with everyday activities and some health care services but typically they do not require 24-hour skilled nursing care services for extended periods of time. The National Center for Assisted Living (NCAL) also emphasizes that these communities offer companionship, independence, and security while prioritizing the choice, dignity, and privacy of residents.

Amenities and Services

Most assisted living residences offer:

- A private or shared room or apartment within a larger residence
- Regular housekeeping, which may or may not include laundry services
- Three meals per day, including snacks and support for some special diets
- Social activities for residents
- Some help with activities of daily living (ADLs), such as bathing, grooming, toileting, transferring in and out of bed or a chair, eating, and continence, though help provided will vary by facility
- Some nursing care, although assisted-living residences are not required to have a registered nurse (RN) on staff

Similar to independent living, assisted living residents enjoy the freedom to come and go as they please. Family and friends can take them out for dinner, shopping, a sporting event, or a family celebration any time—no curfews, no restrictions. Typically, the only requirement is signing the resident out upon departure and back in upon return.

By tracking check-ins and check-outs, staff stay informed, can tailor care to each resident, and ensure everyone is safe and accounted for. For instance, they may provide necessary medications before a resident leaves or follow up upon their return to confirm the latest dose is given.

Beyond the Basics: Comparing Services and Support Levels

Among the differences between independent and assisted living are the degree of support for activities for daily living, staff engagement, and enhanced safety measures. Starting with safety, for example, independent living apartments may have exterior entrances or patios as visitors and residents can come and go at will, whereas, assisted living units typically have interior-facing doors requiring visitors to enter and check in through a central lobby. And exterior doors, whether leading to a covered patio or a driveway, are equipped with chimes that sound whenever someone enters or exits, alerting the staff and ensuring residents' safety, especially those who may experience memory challenges or a tendency to wander off.

Another difference between independent living and assisted living is often seen in the kitchen setup. Assisted living accommodations rarely have an oven or cooktop. Microwave ovens and coffee makers are allowed but baking and cooking in their apartments are prohibited to prevent potential fire hazards, such as forgetting a boiling pot on the stove or leaving the oven on unintentionally.

One kitchen amenity found in independent living and assisted living facilities is a full-size refrigerator-freezer for storing your beverages of choice, which, depending on medical orders, may include beer and wine. After all, this isn't a college dorm. These are adults who have lived full, adventurous lives. They won't be 'written up' by the hall monitor for having alcohol in their refrigerators. For my mom and her perpetual habit of saving, having her own refrigerator is perfect for storing leftovers from every meal she doesn't finish in the dining hall. She's paying for it, so in her mind, 'No need to waste it.'

Along with preventing safety issues, without a fully functioning kitchen, assisted living residents are encouraged to gather in the dining hall for meals. Sharing meals builds community, socialization, and routine. Getting out of the apartment is important for mental and emotional stimulation. It also helps build a routine into an otherwise unstructured string of days. Without some form of a schedule or time commitment, days roll into weeks, weeks into months and with the passing of time, mental and physical decline ensues.

Skilled Nursing, Long-Term Care, and Nursing Home— What are the Differences?

As care needs increase and activities of daily living become more difficult, even with help, assisted living may no longer be enough. When standing and balance are compromised, and lifting or maneuvering requires two people, a move to long-term care often becomes necessary.

The differences between long-term care facilities, skilled nursing facilities, and nursing homes can be confusing, and the terms are often used interchangeably.

To better understand how these facilities differ, each is defined as follows.

Skilled Nursing Facility (SNF)–Skilled nursing facilities are often associated with rehabilitation services, providing intensive medical care for patients who require specialized treatment. For example, after a hospital stay, my mom needed physical therapy (PT) and occupational therapy (OT) to recover from hip surgery. She was discharged from the hospital to a skilled nursing facility, where Medicare covered the facility fees and rehabilitation services. While coverage can vary, Medicare typically pays for up to 21 days of skilled nursing care. After that, additional days may be covered by supplemental insurance policies, if owned or available by private pay arrangements.

One source of confusion is that skilled nursing facilities may exist within a larger long-term care facility or nursing home. A nursing home may have a designated section for patients receiving short-term rehabilitation—staying for just a few weeks rather than residing long term. The difference between a skilled nursing facility and a nursing home is largely based on Medicare regulations, state and federal classifications, and the scope of medical services provided.

Long-Term Care Facility (LTC)—Long-term care facilities support individuals who need help with daily tasks but may not require intensive medical treatment like skilled nursing patients. A key distinction is that skilled nursing facility patients typically receive PT, OT, and speech therapy, with Medicare covering their stay as part of their recovery. Long-term care residents, on the other hand, require ongoing support with activities of daily living but not receiving therapy. Medicare does not cover long-term care costs. Residents pay through private pay funds or, sometimes, through Medicaid or veterans' benefits. Some experts contend that long-term care is not limited to a specific setting but rather refers to the type of services an individual needs. Some use the phrase long-term care to refer to services offered in various settings, including nursing homes, assisted living facilities, and even in individuals' own homes.

Nursing Home Facility–Nursing home facilities typically serve individuals with chronic conditions and offer a residential setting rather than a hospital-like environment. As a result of their similarities, since the terms long-term care and nursing home overlap, they are often used interchangeably.

The term "nursing home" can carry a negative connotation, evoking images of a clinical, institutional setting. "Long-term care facility" is more commonly accepted, as it feels neutral and less stigmatized. Regardless of terminology, both types of facilities provide extended support for individuals with chronic illnesses, disabilities, or limitations in independent living. Services may include help with activities of daily living, medication management, transportation, meal preparation, and emotional support.

Notable physical differences between an assisted living arrangement and a long-term care facility are the room configurations and amenities. Unlike in an assisted living arrangement, the residents have either a private or semi-private room with a bathroom. Bathrooms may not have a designated separation between the shower and toilet. Since residents frequently are non-ambulatory, meaning they can't stand on their own, bathing consists of them sitting in a shower chair as the staff assists or washes them using a shower wand attached to the wall.

Another unique feature of a long-term care facility is a hoist, or a Hoyer lift, which can lift and transfer residents who can no longer stand.

Hoyer lifts provide a safe and efficient way to transfer individuals, reducing the risk of injury for both the patient and the caregiver. Whether it's in a hospital, nursing home, or at home, these lifts ensure transfers are smooth and comfortable.

MEMORY CARE

Another specialized or alternative facility to assisted or independent living is memory care. Memory care units provide a structured and secure environment for individuals experiencing memory loss, particularly those with Alzheimer's disease or other forms of dementia. These units exist within larger senior living facilities or as standalone centers, offering specialized care designed to enhance cognitive function and overall well-being.

Memory care is a form of residential long-term care that provides intensive, 24-hour support for older adults with dementia. Residents benefit from trained staff, tailored activities, and therapies aimed at stimulating memory and engagement. Depending on the facility, memory care units may be independent centers or designated, secured wings within a broader senior living community.

To promote cognitive function and engagement, memory care facilities offer activities such as art and music therapy, which cater to residents at various stages of dementia or Alzheimer's. Since individuals with dementia are prone to wandering, according to the Alzheimer's Association, memory care facilities implement safety measures like alarmed doors, access-controlled elevators, and enclosed outdoor spaces to ensure residents remain within the facility while maintaining a sense of independence.

Planning for the Price Tag: Navigating Costs, Insurance and VA Benefits

Just as the level of care changes across various living facilities, so too do the costs. Research shows that the costs associated with each option vary depending on location, amenities, inflation and supply and demand. One thing is for certain, the more services and assistance with activities of daily living become necessary, costs increase. As a result, assisted living tends to be more expensive than independent living; long-term care is typically more costly than assisted living, and memory care can be even pricier than long-term care.

Some facilities offer a tiered pricing structure, where the greater the resident's needs, the higher the tier of services required, and the lesser the resident's needs, the lower the tier level and the lesser the cost.

Regardless of whether living in an independent dwelling, assisted living facility, or long-term community, Medicare does not cover housing costs. Skilled nursing care is one of the few scenarios in which Medicare covers facility expenses.

According to the National Council on Aging (NCOA), Medicaid likewise does not pay for room and board in independent living and assisted living facilities—two significant expenses that contribute to the overall cost of assisted living. However, there are programs and expenses that Medicaid can help cover. Check with state specific websites to learn about Medicaid waiver programs such as Home and Community-Based Services (HCBS) waivers or 1915(c) Medicaid waivers. These programs help cover various services and support for older adults.

Additionally, some states offer Medicaid-funded long-term care facility programs. To determine eligibility, check with your state's Medicaid office or inquire directly with facilities you're considering whether they accept Medicaid and what the application process entails.

Another option that may be available is veterans' benefits. Veterans may have access to long-term care assistance through the Veterans Administration, provided they require skilled nursing care or help with daily activities. A service-connected disability is not required to qualify. Eligibility depends on factors such as income level, medical needs, and any existing service-related disabilities. Veterans and their families can explore long-term care options by reaching out to a VA social worker or visiting their local VA Medical Center. These benefits support veterans in maintaining their quality of life and independence.

Long-Term Care Insurance—What to Know

This is not legal or financial advice. Consult a certified advisor to explore solutions and options specific to your situation.

When planning for long-term care, one important consideration is long-term care (LTC) insurance, a private insurance option available to those who can afford it. LTC insurance helps cover the cost of nursing-home care, home-health care, and personal or adult daycare for individuals aged 65 or older or those with chronic or disabling conditions requiring ongoing supervision. While it often covers assisted living facilities, there are key limitations to be aware of.

Key Considerations for LTC Insurance

Long-term care insurance rarely covers independent living. However, it can help reduce costs in an independent living community by covering personal care services, meal preparation, housekeeping, and transportation.

There are important stipulations associated with LTC insurance, including:

Benefit triggers–Specific criteria must be met before a policy covers assisted living costs. Like other insurance types, LTC insurance requires policyholders to meet certain benefit triggers before payments begin. This often includes:

- **The inability to perform two of six activities of daily living** without assistance, such as bathing, dressing, or eating.

- **Cognitive impairment**, such as Alzheimer's or dementia, preventing independent living.

Elimination (waiting) periods—Before benefits are paid, policyholders must first satisfy a waiting period, often 30, 60, or 90 days, depending on the policy.

Coverage duration—Policies may provide coverage for a set time frame, typically two to five years. Some policies offer unlimited coverage, though these are less common. Most LTC policies have a maximum duration of coverage. For example, a policy with a $500 daily benefit and a two-year coverage limit may fully cover assisted living costs for those two years. However, after that period, the individual must seek alternative payment methods if they remain in assisted living.

If you already own or are considering purchasing a long-term care insurance policy, understanding its limitations—particularly regarding assisted living, independent living, and Medicare exclusions—is crucial in making informed decisions.

Source: Does Long-Term Care Insurance Cover Assisted Living? - ElderLife Financial

UNDERSTANDING THE NUMBERS—COST DIFFERENCES BY FACILITY TYPE

The cost of senior living facilities continues to rise because of increasing demand due to the growing aging population. To navigate these expenses and create a financial strategy for your aging parents' retirement, consulting a financial planner is highly recommended.

For reference, according to a Genworth CareScout study, here are some estimated costs for long-term care in 2024:

- **Aging in Place (Home Health Aide):** The average annual cost for home health aide services was $78,000, based on 44 hours per week for 52 weeks a year.

- **Assisted Living Community:** The national median annual cost for assisted living was $70,000, reflecting a 10 percent increase from the previous year, with occupancy rates rising from 77 percent to 84 percent.

- **Private Room Nursing Home:** The median annual cost for a private nursing home room was $127,750, marking a 9 percent increase over the previous year, based 365 days of care.

With costs steadily rising, proactive financial planning is essential to ensure the best possible care options for aging loved ones.

SO MANY OPTIONS—WHAT'S RIGHT FOR MOM?

Every aging parent's needs are different, and understanding the distinctions between various facilities, their amenities, and when a particular option may be suitable at one stage, but perhaps not throughout the entire journey, is essential. Here is a helpful checklist to consider when researching senior care facilities.

Research and Understand Your Options

Learn about senior care options-explore the different types of care available.

Understand health care services-review medical care, specialized therapies, and health and safety protocols.

Assess Needs and Preferences

Consider care needs-determine the level of support required.

Consider your loved one's preferences-factor in lifestyle choices and personal comfort.

Evaluate Costs and Financial Considerations

Review overall pricing-get a broad understanding of costs across different care levels.

Dig deeper into costs-break down expenses, including hidden or additional fees.

Research and Compare Facilities

Check facility safety records-ensure compliance with regulations and past performance.

Ask about staffing ratios and tenure-learn how well the facility is staffed and employee retention rates.

Ask about emergency protocols-understand how emergencies are handled.

Tour your favorite options-visit top choices to get a firsthand impression.

Assess Daily Living and Amenities

Learn about activities-explore social, recreational, and engagement opportunities.

Discuss transportation-understand mobility options and accessibility.

Try the food-sample meals to gauge quality and variety.

Spoiler alert: Mom doesn't flash a smile, embrace uncertainty, and joyfully agree to leave the home she built with Dad. She doesn't seamlessly transition from her first respite care stay into an independent living community. No, her journey is far more complicated, as I suspect is true for most families. Convincing Mom to leave her home requires patience, creativity, and difficult conversations. With each experience, we learn more, ask better questions, and sharpen our understand of what truly matters.

Educate yourself. Research options. Ask the hard questions.
The more informed you are, the better prepared you'll be to
make crucial decisions before a crisis arises. Knowledge is power,
and preparation eases the weight of urgent decision-making.

CHAPTER 12

Mom Jobs - Managing Mom's Household

Topics

— Tackling "Mom Jobs": Keeping Up with Household Tasks

— Coverage Confusion: Renewing Auto Insurance

— When Monthly Costs Increase: Managing Retirement Account Withdrawals

The list of "Project Mom" tasks feels endless—even when she eventually moves into a senior living facility. Just like my bulk-shopping habits, I try to approach my own household chores with ruthless efficiency: line up all the errands on Saturday, make eleven stops, knock everything out, and get home before dinner. I try managing Mom chores in much the same way. But somehow, no matter how many boxes I check, the to-do list keeps growing.

When we discover Mom's auto insurance is about to be canceled or she's being fined by the HOA for an overgrown lawn, it's clear we need to step in more actively. Managing her life goes far beyond coordinating medical care, hiring support services, or sorting out rehab options. The role of the project manager of Mom's life is expanding. Now, along with caregiver coordination and tending to medical needs, we are also handling everything from financial decision making to home maintenance.

Tackling "Mom Jobs": Keeping Up with Household Tasks

"Project Mom" remains a full-time job—and it's aging me. I've gained thirty pounds in the past two years. The gym has been remodeled since I last stepped foot in it, and my stylist is stocking up on extra hair dye to keep pace with my graying roots.

Every task feels heavy. I've developed a full-blown case of the *I don't want to's*. Nothing specific has changed—just my attitude. But I keep going because I have no other choice.

Today's to-do list includes:

- Resolve her auto insurance coverage
- Increase her monthly retirement withdrawal
- Follow up on lawn care service
- Don't pick a fight with my sister

The tasks are piling up with no finish line in sight.

Recurring Monthly Costs

I tackle the *don't pick a fight with my sister* task first. Tina and I have different approaches when it comes to managing money. Since she oversees Mom's day-to-day expenses, her financial strategies often shape how we approach Mom's household budget. Sometimes this works. Other times it sparks tension.

Take the cable bill. When Tina's rates go up, she pivots to streaming services to save money. Sensible for her, but not for Mom. Streaming platforms are a foreign concept. All she wants is to catch the ten o'clock local news and watch the Cardinals play. *Why change what is working?*

Beyond Mom's preference for local TV, the thought of swapping out a router or changing a service provider introduces a host of unforeseen problems. What if switching providers means losing the telephone number she and Dad have had for years? Their phone number is a single constant that old friends use to keep in touch.

Relying solely on Mom's cell phone might save money, but it isn't practical. The landline gives her reliable access to make and receive calls. It also ensures she can dial 911 in an emergency—no worries about electrical outages.

In the end, Tina and I agree to strip back the TV package to lower costs while minimizing disruption. We avoid unnecessary tech drama, and a fight with my sister is averted.

Coverage Confusion: Renewing Auto Insurance

Task number two on my ever-growing to-do list: renew Mom's auto insurance. Her policy is up for renewal, but there's a hitch—her driver's license has expired, which makes her ineligible for coverage. Selling the minivan isn't an option yet. It's my lifeline when I visit, saving me from rental car fees and logistical headaches. So now I need to find a way to keep the vehicle insured without raising red flags.

Although my best Mom impersonation works fine with the cable company, auto insurance is a different beast. They already know her license is expired, so I have to be honest—identify myself, explain the situation, and hope they'll work with me. And I also need to be careful not to mention her homeowner's policy, which is up for renewal in six months. Tina's warning: if the insurance company finds out no one's living in the house full-time, they might refuse to renew. That is a problem for future us. Right now, the minivan is the priority.

Navigating these calls as Mom's power of attorney is always tricky. Most customer service reps have no clue what POA actually means. It's not part of their training. But this time, I get lucky. The woman who answers understands immediately. She asks me to fax the documents.

Fax? *Who faxes documents anymore, aside from medical practices?* We hang up; I scan the required documents and attach them to an email.

To my surprise, the agent calls me back within ten minutes. She's now 'officially' allowed to speak with me. I explain that Mom is in a senior living facility and can't drive. And just like that, the conversation pivots. "So, your mother isn't living in her home. She has homeowner insurance coverage with us." *Oh dear Lord. Can we just stay focused on renewing the auto insurance? Have I tripped a wire? Is a bigger issue unfolding?*

"We are talking about the auto policy," I say.

"Yes, but she also has her homeowner policy with us."

I ask when the homeowner policy is up for renewal, and she says October.

"Okay. So we've got six months before we need to address that, yes?"

"Yes. But we need to know if she's living there."

"She is getting better and plans to return to her home," I lie. "And I visit and stay in the house a couple of weeks each month." Another lie. "Can we please focus on the auto insurance?"

You may be able to renew a homeowner's insurance policy online. Simply set up an account, add a form of online payment such as a credit card, and the policy will auto renew—no questions asked.

The conversation with the rep continues. She hesitates and says, "Her auto policy is expiring and won't be renewed."

I ask how we can get it renewed and if I can be added to the policy. She tells me we need to sell the car.

"No. We are not selling the car." I raise my voice. "Can you add me to the policy?" She tells me we need to carry insurance on the vehicle. *No kidding. Why else would I be talking to you?* Then, she asks if I have a valid driver's license, and I confirm I do.

"Are you insured?" she asks.

"Yes." *Now we are getting somewhere. I've got a driver's license. I carry auto insurance. We're making progress.*

She tells me she needs to talk to her underwriter and will get back to me. A few hours pass, and the agent calls back and says she can't add me to the policy. When I press for the reason, she becomes agitated and says, "This is a very complicated case. The policy cannot be renewed."

When I ask if she can write a new policy, we go through the same set of questions: do I have a driver's license and am I insured? *For God's sake.*

"Well, I'll need to get you over to our new coverage department. I'm unable to help you."

"Okay. Send me over." Now I'm the one who is frustrated.

"I'm patching you over to Quanita. She'll take care of you."

"Thank you, Marcia. You've been a great help." *No, she hasn't. She's not done a darn thing for me but waste my day.*

"This is Quanita. How may I help you?"

"Hi Quanita. Has Marcia briefed you on my situation?"

"Yes. I understand you want a quote for a new policy."

Quanita asks for my driver's license number.

"Okay. I live in Texas. My license number is…"

Quanita interrupts. "Oh lordy. You don't live in Missouri?"

"No,"

"Is the car in Missouri?"

"Yes,"

"Is the car abandoned?"

"No. It is in the garage."

"Who lives in the house?" *Oh God. Here we go again.*

"Where do you want the car to be?" I concede. *It can be parked at my sister's house. It can be in my mom's garage. Wherever you want the car to be, it will be there.*

"You see. I can't write this policy because you live out of state."

My voice quivers. "Quanita. I don't mean to be rude, but I've been at this all day. I just need to get this car insured. I have a mother with a disability. I need a vehicle to drive when I'm in town. Can you please help me?"

"I understand, but I have to do this legally. You don't want me to do it illegally now, do you?"

My patience expires. "No. I'm not asking you to break the rules, but you need to show me some empathy. I've been at this all day and I'm no closer to having it resolved."

Quanita course corrects. She acknowledges my exasperation and says, "Honey. I understand. My father is ninety years old, and he too, lives out of state. Let's see what we can do for you." *Finally, a reasonable human.*

Quanita and I are on the same page. She understands my plight and genuinely wants to help me problem-solve. We work through options and determine that ultimately Tina must be the auto insurance policyholder, since she lives in the state where the vehicle resides. We can park in Tina's garage, and I'll be an authorized driver of the vehicle. *Success!*

Quanita continues, "I just need to talk to your sister. I need her driver's license information."

And just like that, my day-long task ends with me running face-first into a brick wall. I can't close the action on my to-do list; I feel defeated.

Depleted, but appreciative of Quanita's compassion, I thank her and hang up. I compose an email, document the details, include Quanita's number and turn the case over to Tina to resolve.

Tina is compassionate and helpful. She empathizes with my ordeal and willingly picks up the ball. Two days later, I receive an email from her. "Done. I renewed the policy. You are insured to drive the vehicle, and the lady I talked to said, 'Your sister was really upset. I wished I could have helped her.' I know how frustrating this must have been for you. Thanks for taking this on."

Mom Job—Deal with Lawn Treatment

As much as I'd like to work through my *project plan* and mark every project milestone as 100 percent complete in a single day—or even a week—Mom tasks seldom work that way. As soon as one task is cleared, another pops up.

Next up: renewing Mom's lawn treatment service. The goal is simple—keep the weeds at bay, avoid neighbor complaints, and, most importantly, stay off the HOA's radar. I call the lawn care company, review the seasonal treatment schedule, confirm they still have a credit card on file, and hang up.

Done. A clean, easy win.

With the yard maintenance officially on autopilot for the year, I feel a small surge of relief. One less thing to worry about. That quick success gives me just enough momentum to face the harder tasks still ahead.

When Monthly Costs Increase: Managing Retirement Account Withdrawals

The next task on my to-do list: managing Mom's retirement investments and making sure her monthly withdrawals cover her needs.

When my husband, Rick, and I were newly married, he cautiously agreed to help my parents oversee their retirement savings. He's skilled at investment planning, but it's not his profession, and as the new son-in-law, he didn't want to overstep.

Despite his initial reluctance, Rick's strategic vision and thoughtful planning kept Mom's finances stable. Her savings continued to support her needs, and we were incredibly fortunate. Thanks to his smart investing and fiscal discipline, Mom has the financial foundation to sustain her care.

After Dad passed, Rick willingly stepped back, and the responsibility of managing Mom's retirement finances shifted to me. I've always understood the value of contributing to a retirement plan, ever since my first job.

Now, I'm navigating the other side of the equation: the art of drawing funds out. It's a different kind of financial literacy—one that requires just as much strategy, but with a sharper focus on sustainability and care. I face yet another self-directed learning exercise—Required Mandatory Distribution.

For detailed guidance, always consult a tax adviser. But here's the gist—once someone reaches a certain age (which shifts as tax laws evolve), they're required to withdraw a minimum amount each year from retirement accounts like IRAs. Because these funds were contributed pre-tax, withdrawals are taxable. How much must be withdrawn annually is calculated based on the account's value at the end of the previous calendar year.

Bottom line: Mom is obligated to take out a set amount each year and pay taxes on it. She can choose to withdraw the full amount in one lump sum or spread it out in monthly installments. Either way, it's one more financial lever I need to manage carefully.

After my Dad passed, Mom clung tightly to her frugal instincts. Despite gentle nudging from my sister and me to ease up and use their retirement savings to support a more comfortable lifestyle, she refused to budge. Living within her means was a point of pride. She saw it as a challenge, and she met it head-on by relying solely on her monthly Social Security checks.

At first, her approach held up. But now as her health declines and her needs grow, those checks no longer stretch far enough. We now must bridge the gap by drawing monthly funds from her IRA.

Seniors without savings often combine public programs, part-time work, housing changes, and community support to sustain themselves.

KEY ALTERNATIVES FOR SENIORS WITHOUT ADEQUATE SAVINGS

Social Security and Public Benefits

- Social Security remains the primary income source for many retirees.

- Supplemental Security Income (SSI) can help those with very limited resources.

- Medicaid may cover long-term care costs, while Medicare provides health coverage.

Part-Time or Flexible Work

- Many seniors continue working part-time to supplement income.

Housing Adjustments

- Downsizing to a smaller home or apartment reduces expenses.

- Shared housing or multigenerational living arrangements can cut costs and provide companionship.

- Some communities offer subsidized senior housing.

Community and Nonprofit Resources

- Local senior centers often provide meals, transportation, and social activities.

- Charities and nonprofits may help with utility bills, food, or medical costs.

- Faith-based organizations sometimes offer caregiving support.

Healthcare and Insurance Planning

- Medicaid can cover nursing home or in-home care for those with limited assets.

- Medicare Advantage or supplemental plans may reduce out-of-pocket medical costs.

Lifestyle Adjustments

- Practice careful budgeting, debt reduction, and prioritizing essential expenses.

- Consider moving to lower-cost regions or countries where living expenses are more manageable.

SPENDING ACCELERATES WITH AGE

Experts often describe retirement spending in three phases. In early retirement years, spending starts high with travel and leisure, dips in the middle, and often rises again in the final phase due to healthcare and caregiving costs. Expenses like assisted living, in-home care, and long-term skilled nursing can quickly accelerate the drawdown of savings. Put simply, the older we get, the faster we tend to burn through retirement funds.

When Mom eventually moves into a long-term care facility full time, her savings begin to shrink at an alarming rate. Daily room and board fees keep climbing, driving her annual expenses up by more than 10 percent.

This increase means I must recalibrate her monthly withdrawals. Tina needs enough in the checking account to cover ongoing household expenses, since we're still maintaining Mom's home. On paper, keeping the house seems impractical. Financially, it's hard to justify. But emotionally, I'm not ready to let it go, and keeping the house gives me a place to stay for the many weeks when I'm in town.

To Mom, the house is more than bricks and mortar. It represents her life's work, her greatest accomplishment, and in her eyes, her most valuable asset. Selling it before she passes feels like a betrayal—like erasing a part of her identity while she's still here. For now, the house stays. It's the one tangible piece of her story she can still hold onto.

Springing for Additional Services

When it comes to spending Mom's money, my sister and I do not always see eye to eye. As with many things, she and I approach the situation differently. Neither of us is acting from a position of greed or selfishness. We both subscribe to the idea of 'last dollar, last breath.' In other words, whatever financial reserves Mom has, they are there to provide for her needs.

Our differences stem from how Tina and I live, and how we make decisions. For example, if Mom needs a new wheelchair and Medicare declines the claim because she permanently lives in a skilled nursing facility (a seemingly broken process in the medical system), then I have no problem using her resources to pay for the equipment. Sure, I'd like Medicare to cover it, but if we question it and they refuse, I let it go. Mom needs the wheelchair. She has the money. From my perspective, we buy her the equipment and close the 'task.' Our time, effort, and stress in fighting with Medicare takes more effort than I'm willing or able to expend.

Tina, on the other hand, sees this problem twofold. One, she wants to honor Mom's wishes and squeeze every penny. The thought of paying out-of-pocket for a piece of equipment that *should* be covered *violates* Mom's financial code. And two, the fact that Medicare refuses to cover the cost of this much-needed device is an injustice in the eyes of both my mother and my sister.

Although both may be correct (the wheelchair should be a covered expense), I believe if Mom needs the device and she has the funds to pay for it, we should buy it. Wasting time and energy fighting the system feels futile. I am confident we are staying vigilant in managing Mom's finances while keeping her needs top of mind. *Maybe I need to re-visit my don't pick a fight with your sister task.*

Another area where Tina and I clash over funding Mom's needs is the topic of providing additional companion care at the skilled nursing facility. Mom has an insatiable need for human interaction and conversation. In my opinion, she can benefit from a companion caregiver who will sit with her in the evenings as she relaxes and gets ready for bed. To me, if this helps soothe her nerves and brings her peace, it's worth hiring someone for a few hours each night. Although the staff can visit with Mom for short periods of time, they have other residents to attend to.

What frustrates Tina is that when all residents have been attended, the staff doesn't go above and beyond. When they are available to return to Mom's room and sit with her for an hour, they instead 'relax' and 'check out.' I admit that from our perspective, it would be nice if they optimized their time, but they don't. And to be fair, we don't fully know what other responsibilities they have outside of tending to residents' needs. They might need to complete charts, prepare meals for the next day, or handle other behind-the-scenes tasks.

While Tina believes the staff should be 'earning their keep,' I see things differently. If Mom is safe, cared for, clean and eating regularly, I'm good. The facility and staff are caring for her in ways we can't, and for that I am grateful. Sitting with Mom, keeping her company isn't the staff's responsibility—it's ours.

If we can't be there as often as Mom wants, or simply don't have the bandwidth, then the answer is clear: we hire someone to sit with her. To listen. To be present.

In spite of how differently Tina and I approach things, at the core, we're aligned. We're committed to the same mission: caring for Mom with dignity and compassion as she ages. We both want what's best for her, and that helps us get past the bumps and keeps us moving forward.

RESOURCES

Required Minimum Distribution (RMD) Calculator (aarp.org)

CHAPTER 13

Building a Support Network

Topics

— Building Your Circle: Creating a Support System

— Leaning In: Tapping Family, Friends, and Trusted Confidants

— Digital Lifelines: Leveraging Online Communities and Resources

— Old Ties, New Strength: Reconnecting with Childhood Friends and Former Neighbors

Raise your hand if your aging parent still uses the White Pages from 2010 or if their tattered phone book has pages falling out? Well, I quit making fun of my mom's forty-year-old vintage phone book when it became my lifeline. Neighbors, friends, distant relatives, these names and numbers are golden.

Caring for an aging parent is a journey that tests us, and having a support system isn't just helpful, it's essential. A support system includes people who can relate to what we are going through, people who I can complain to, cry in front of and who don't judge me. They offer tips and recommendations as an elder parent transitions from one stage of the aging process to the next. High school social media connections and friends from the 'old neighborhood' are great resources as childhood friends offer a perspective of what Mom was like when I was growing up. While she may now be a frail shell of her former self, hometown friends may remember her as vibrant and active. She was their beloved Girl Scout leader or the nice lunchroom lady who put an extra cookie on their tray.

As valuable as it is reconnecting with those who knew Mom in the past, building relationships with her current friends and neighbors is also helpful. If Mom plays bridge, attends a Silver Sneakers exercise class, socializes with neighbors, or belongs to a Bible study, get to know her social circle. These everyday connections with an aging parent can offer perspective if Mom doesn't seem "quite right." They can recommend doctors they've used and facilities to consider along with a list of the ones to avoid. Other helpful resources include websites, social media platforms and professional connections.

Building Your Circle: Creating a Support System

Caring for an aging parent is hard. I find myself watching my Mom lose more and more independence each day. The toll is heavy on me and on those who love me. It infiltrates my life in ways I never imagined, and the hardest part is not knowing how long this role will last. It could be weeks, months, or years. The uncertainty is overwhelming, often showing up as exhaustion, depression, or other health issues. It strains relationships too. Though invisible to others, the pressure weighs on me daily. That's why I try prioritizing my own well-being and lean on a strong support system. I'm not always successful. In fact, I probably fail at it more than achieve it, but I try surrounding myself with friends, family, and resources I can reach out to for help.

One of the most pivotal lessons I've learned is the power of social networks. Don't be afraid to reach out and connect. I may call someone I talk to regularly or ping a distant acquaintance on social media. Asking for a recommendation or advice can turn into a much-needed lifeline. A support system can be a spouse, adult children, close friends, a spiritual advisor, or a therapist, anyone who is trustworthy and reliable. Beyond my inner circle, Mom's medical staff, physical and occupational therapists, and doctors are also critical resources.

Each resource, whether personal or professional, can be a guide when making decisions about a loved one's care. As I navigate Mom's journey, I always save in my phone directory the names and contact information of helpful individuals I meet along the way. I never know when I might need to call on them in the future.

Hold onto familiar, healthy routines that help center you. If you attend a weekly Bible study, regularly practice yoga, take daily walks, or indulge in a mani/pedi, keep making time for things that ground you. These small yet significant anchors foster self-care and provide stability amidst the challenges of caring for an aging parent. Remember, perfection isn't the goal. And although it may not be possible every day, try to prioritize your own well-being the best you can.

LEANING ON FAMILY

Caring for an aging parent can sometimes push relationships to their breaking point. I've seen it firsthand. A close friend's thirty-year marriage ended because of the overwhelming stress that came with caregiving, which can be an all-consuming responsibility, often unbearable. No matter how much I want to stay present in my "real life"—the one with my spouse, my children and my job, I find myself distracted, consumed by worry. *Will Mom fall again? Was my last trip the last time I'll see her alive? What if, while I'm traveling for work or on a family vacation, I get the dreaded call that she's back in the hospital and I have to catch the next flight out?*

I'm fortunate to have a loving partner and two incredibly supportive children. With every frantic trip to the airport, I leave behind a wake of chaos; laundry left undone, barren pantry shelves and a nearly empty bag of dog food. Yet, my husband and sons step in without hesitation, meeting the plumber scheduled to fix a leaky faucet or getting my car in for its much overdue oil change.

But while they willingly pick up the pieces, they, too, grow weary. The loose ends I drop don't disappear; someone else has to manage them. Once or twice, they understand, but this has become our new reality. We're all exhausted, stretched thin, questioning how much longer we can live in this chaos, this uncertainty—this hell. And as difficult as it is, it's essential to extend grace and forgiveness, both to others and to ourselves.

An Excerpt from a Friend

For almost seventeen years, I took care of my husband's mom and grandmother. They were sweet, petite little Italian ladies prone to moments of piss and vinegar and the extreme emotions that cultural stereotypes propagate.

One of the most memorable moments was great-grandma's quick descent into the depths of grief when someone she knew died. Like Scarlet O'Hara, she would raise an arm across her eyes and bemoan the fact that it should have been her that had gone to meet her maker rather than the person who'd been so lucky as to sneak into the afterlife before her. She'd been trying to die for years, and as one year passed into another to bring her closer to her centennial birthday, I'm sure she was ready.

Most days it was easy to find humor in her antics, but there were plenty of others, when the burdens of caretaking weighed heavily on my shoulders, that I wondered what she was waiting for. Secretly, I felt caring for her was stealing the best years of my young adulthood, my parenting and my marriage, and I became entangled in shame that I could wish for her to die.

And so it continued. Awaken each day with a new determination. Close each day huddled on the floor of the shower, sobbing from exhaustion on every level possible. I didn't know I could or should be asking for help.

SIBLING CIVILITY

Extending grace to siblings can often be one of the most challenging aspects of partnering in the care of an aging parent. In my family, brothers approach conflict with less emotion and more pragmatism. I saw this firsthand with my husband and his brothers when they cared for their dying father. When my father-in-law entered hospice, each brother pulled out his calendar, assigned himself a weekend and executed the plan without argument or negotiation. One brother took the lead during the week, communicated updates and made decisions when necessary. If disagreements arose, they talked it through calmly until deciding to stick with or adjust the plan. That was their reality, though I'm certain not all families experience male sibling dynamics quite this smoothly.

Sister relationships, however, seem to carry a greater likelihood of friction. This isn't exactly new wisdom. Sayings like, "No house is big enough for two women" date back to ancient times. Whether because of personality differences, passion, temperament, or pent-up expectations regarding roles and responsibilities, sisters fight. Whatever the motivation, sharing caregiving responsibilities with a sibling can be difficult.

My sister and I have always had a love/hate relationship. Some days we get along effortlessly; other days, it feels like we can't stand each other. We approach communication, problem-solving and decision-making differently. We lead vastly different lives. My sister is a single parent who lives ten miles from Mom's house, while I'm married with two kids, living 600 miles away in Texas.

We disagree on just about everything from politics to child rearing. We disagree on handling finances. We disagree about so many things that when it comes to working together to solve problems or negotiating how to handle Mom issues; it takes tremendous effort on both sides.

Over the ten years we've partnered to manage Mom's care, my sister and I have had countless arguments. Feelings have been hurt, and tempers have flared. But we keep talking. We keep communicating. This isn't easy, but we make the choice to move forward. We don't always agree with the decisions the other one makes, but we keep striving to do what is best for Mom. Despite our differences, we share a common goal: ensuring Mom receives the care and support she deserves.

Leaning In: Tapping Family, Friends, and Trusted Confidants

Beyond family, others are available to help and support. Don't hesitate to ask for help, offer a return favor, and embrace the opportunity to connect. Mom's neighbors are a Godsend. As she comes and goes with a 'broken hip' here, and a 'respite care stay' there, neighbors keep watch over her house, retrieve the mail and ensure flyers don't pile up at the front door. If a sprinkler head is misbehaving or a spring storm brings heavy rain and wind, we get a text. "The house is good. Doesn't look like there is any damage."

I make it a point to say hello to the neighbors when I'm in town and ensure we have each other's contact information. They are curious and concerned, always interested in how things are going. One neighbor, coincidentally, also has parents who live about thirty miles from me in Texas. We instantly connect, sharing worries and woes of caring for aging parents across state lines. We swap stories and share resources on everything from 'When do you bring a caregiver into their home' to 'Have you checked out any skilled nursing centers nearby?' Whenever this neighbor sees Mom's van in the driveway (the one I drive when I visit), I get a text, "You in town?" And an instant friendship is born.

STAYING CONNECTED AS MOM'S HEALTH DETERIORATES

As Mom's health continues to decline, eventually requiring her to move into a long-term care facility, feelings of hopelessness and isolation naturally set in. Her neighbors remain loyal. They ask about her often and stop by her facility for a visit from time to time.

One Valentine's Day, the facility sponsored a Sweetheart Message event, inviting friends and family to send roses or candygrams to the residents. I sent out a group text to rally support. The message went to all the neighbors and my parents' lifelong friends who live out of state. The responses I received were incredible. Everyone wanted to show their love and remind Mom she was cherished and remembered. By the end of the day, her room was filled with a vase of silk roses and enough Valentine's candy to last through the summer.

People genuinely want to help. They just need to be asked. While building my own support system is crucial, it is equally important that

Mom has one too. Reminding her that friends, neighbors and caregivers-turned-family love and care for her brings her comfort. And their compassion helps me replenish my ever-depleting emotional reserves, allowing me to keep showing up for her.

Digital Lifelines: Leveraging Online Communities and Resources

Leveraging online connections is powerful. Although I no longer reside in St. Louis, where Mom is, many of my social media connections still live in the area. Once when we were in need of a new in-home caregiver, I took to social media for recommendations. I posted a request to all my St. Louis connections.

> *St. Louis friends — I'm looking for premium-quality elder care for in-home support. We've had many, many test runs, and only one caregiver has truly met our expectations.*
> *Please DM me if you have a resource. I'm not looking for a company to do a search. Already got that going (two companies in fact...) but I'm looking for a rock star.*

The comments poured in, ranging from heartfelt prayers and empathetic messages to promising leads that turned into interviews and one caregiver who eventually becomes Mom's next in-home companion. One friend even offered to fly to St. Louis and sit with my mom for a few days! Friends want to help, so let them. Although I don't do it perfectly, I try to find the courage to be vulnerable and ask for what I need. I'm often surprised by the outpouring of support.

Old Ties, New Strength: Reconnecting with Childhood Friends and Former Neighbors

During one of Mom's many hospital visits (when she broke her other hip), we opted to have her recover in a specialized rehab facility as opposed to being in a skilled nursing center. This type of dedicated facility is generally for stroke patients and those with severe head injuries, but it appealed to us because we believed the vigorous treatment would have her back on her feet quickly. I explained to Mom the rigor and intense physical therapy patients undergo at this facility, and she was immediately onboard. She was excited. Mom never backs down from a physical challenge. Athleticism is her superpower. With this in mind, we contacted the intake coordinator, who evaluated her and determined she was a perfect fit and off she went to hip-rehab, bootcamp style.

The facility and staff did not disappoint. In just three short weeks, Mom was on her feet, walking with a cane and needing minimal assistance. I was so impressed with her rehab team and how quickly she recovered, I even wrote a review–something I rarely do.

> *Excellent facility. Excellent patient care. My mother has been in two rehab facilities in 12 months. Two separate incidents, both broken hips. The last rehab facility was good; Mercy is exceptional. Clean, quality, professional staff. Physicians listen to the patient and the family for input. PT is great, pleasant, professional, experienced and encouraging. Mom's case manager is the best I've ever worked with. She's detail-oriented, communicative, professional and flexible. She does the job you always hope a case manager will do but rarely have I experienced it. Thanks for the love, support and care in supporting my mother's journey back to independence.*

Months after I posted the review, an old high school friend, someone I hadn't connected with in years, reached out through social media. What started as a few casual messages about the rehab facility soon grew into a phone call, rekindling a long-lost friendship that has since become incredibly special to me. It's amazing to think that writing a simple review about Mom's stay could spark such a meaningful connection.

Robin and I first met in junior high school. Although we didn't know each other's mothers back then, we lived just a few miles apart. Over the years, we both moved away from where we grew up. Robin settled in a suburb west of St. Louis, while I now live in the Dallas-Fort Worth area.

Despite the distance and time, there's a deep, intrinsic connection between us. Robin has become a trusted companion. As Mom's debilitating neuropathy progresses and the stress of managing her care becomes increasingly overwhelming, Robin is always there to listen with understanding and empathy. Our conversations are a judgement free zone where I can be completely open, and she truly gets it. She's living a similar reality, juggling the demands of a full-time job, grown children, and the relentless fatigue that comes with caring for an aging parent. Our exchanges are raw, honest and profoundly comforting—a sisterhood. I'm endlessly grateful. We share our frustrations about navigating a broken healthcare system, the tension and conflicts that arise with our sisters, and the heavy burden of wondering how long we can endure this life of uncertainty.

Along with emotional support, Robin and I often exchange resources and recommendations. It's common for our conversations, whether by phone or text, to begin with insights like, "I just learned Medicare now covers..." or advice tips such as, "I wouldn't put Mom there; the social worker isn't helpful, the staff-to-patient ratio is off; they have high turnover."

As fate will have it, our moms eventually end up at the same long-term care facility. The ladies meet for the first time and share a mutual love of dogs. Along with getting to know Robin's mom, Milly, my mom also meets Snickers, Milly's dog, who visits the facility often. Snickers brings unconditional affection to all the residents, a great thing for the elders, yet one more stressor for Robin as the pooch's permanent home is now with Robin and her husband.

Don't underestimate the value of childhood friends and former neighbors. Even if you have not spoken in years, reach out. Sharing a past together often means these connections might be going through similar life events—experiences you can relate to and understand together.

DOING THE BEST YOU CAN

Keep moving forward, one step at a time. I've learned that I'm not expected to have all the answers, and it's natural to question the choices I make along the caregiver journey. Just as I sometimes look back and wish I had done some things differently when raising children, I remind myself that in each moment, I make the best decision I can with the information I have. The same holds true for caregiving.

Whether navigating this alone as an only child or sharing responsibilities with siblings, I remind myself to seek grace and forgiveness. Building a support system of friends and professionals is invaluable—it's a source of strength that can help lighten the load. And while asking for help may feel like the hardest part, it's often the most important lesson this journey can teach us.

RESOURCES

Along with friends and extended relationships, also consider searching for online resources.

Senior Lifestyle - *www.seniorlifestyle.com* - 40 Resources for Adult Children Caring For Aging Parents Lifestyle

Senior Lifestyle - *www.seniorlifestyle.com* - 7 Signs of Caregiver Burnout

Where You Live Matters - *www.whereyoulivematters.org* - Tips for Long-Distance Caregiving | Where You Live Matters

Taking Care of YOU: Self-Care for Family Caregivers

Caregiving with Your Siblings - Family Caregiver Alliance

Francine Russo on Managing Sibling Relationships in the Caregiving Process

Francine Russo on Managing Sibling Relationships in the Caregiving Process—YouTube Video

CHAPTER 14

The Ruse:
Moving Into Assisted Living

Topics

— Appealing to the Head, Heart and Hands to Guide Change

— Better Safe than Sorry-Accept the Ambulance Ride

— "While You Recover"- Temporary Words, a Permanent Stay

— Two Truths: Her Decline, My Quiet Aching

Helping a reluctant elder transition into assisted living takes compassion and, often, a bit of creativity. In our case, the need for change became clear as Mom's falls and emergency room visits grew more frequent. Her latest trip to the ER becomes a natural pivot point for moving her to a safer, more supportive environment.

It is all about positioning. Whether I am serving up an idea to a business client or trying to get my kids on board with something they don't want to do, it comes down to how I frame the idea. To get Mom to do something she doesn't want to, we use thoughtful language that can ease her resistance, saying things like, "This is temporary, just while you're recovering," to reduce anxiety and preserve dignity. We keep conversations gentle, hopeful, and forward-looking. With the right tone and timing, even difficult transitions can unfold with less friction and more grace.

Appealing to the Head, Heart and Hands to Guide Change

Mom always said, "Never lie." But sometimes, bending the truth becomes a form of mercy. Caring for a resistant aging parent demands creative problem-solving, much like wrangling a defiant first grader or navigating a dysfunctional team at work. When safety is at stake, drastic measures aren't just justified; they're necessary. Getting Mom out of her home and into assisted living is one of these moments.

What started as a manageable caregiving role has morphed into full-blown "scope creep," as the business world calls it. The demands keep growing. Mom can no longer live alone safely, and the situation now calls for expanded resources: increased staff, nurses, a care team, a social director, a dietician, and a facility equipped to meet her developing needs.

ADDING A DOSE OF CHANGE MANAGEMENT

The biggest hurdle isn't logistics; it's emotion. Mom's intense need for control, paired with a paralyzing fear of change, creates a toxic resistance to receiving help. To navigate this, I've had to reach for every change management tool I use in my professional life. Only now, the stakes are personal.

A guiding principle in change management is the "head, heart, and hands" framework. The head speaks to logic, reason, and data—the analytical case for change. The heart focuses on emotional resonance and motivation, helping clarify why the change matters. The hands represent action: removing obstacles and smoothing the path forward. When friction is reduced, transitions become more natural and sustainable.

Navigating Care with an Empath

Along with Mom's deep fear of change, she embodies the traits of an empath, someone who feels the emotional undercurrents around her with startling intensity. An empath can sense and feel another's emotions. They have heightened awareness of all their surroundings, everything from room furnishings to people to animals and nature. And, sometimes an empath can in fact *feel* emotion around them, essentially "absorbing" it, taking on a feeling as their own.

If Mom senses that a care team member is insincere, or if she senses their annoyance with her, she'll resist, sometimes passively, sometimes aggressively.

This sensitivity, paired with her fierce attachment to familiar spaces and routines, makes the idea of leaving her home nearly unthinkable. Logic doesn't land. Reason doesn't persuade. The decision to move her into assisted living cannot be hers—at least not in the traditional sense. It has to be made on her behalf, with compassion and strategy.

This is not easy. There's no comfort in bending the truth, but it's become necessary. The reality she clings to no longer matches the risks she faces. The hard conversations have happened about aging, about the house, about safety. She's fallen, rehabbed, and bounced back more times than anyone can count. At this point, she's earned elite status at the local ER. And the promise to keep her in her home as long as possible has run its course. Now, the priority shifts to keeping her safe, even if it means rewriting the narrative to help her accept the change.

Better Safe than Sorry-Accept the Ambulance Ride

Mom's most recent fall happened with a caregiver nearby. As she stepped out of the bathroom, her jacket snagged on a doorknob, pulling her off balance. She lost her footing and went down hard. The caregiver called 911 immediately, then phoned me. While paramedics were enroute, I opened the mobile app connected to the kitchen cameras to livestream the situation.

Normally, I don't eavesdrop through the cameras because the dialogue between Mom and her caregivers is theirs to share. Respecting her privacy is part of maintaining trust. But this time is different. I need to see and hear what is going on among Mom, the caregiver and the paramedics.

When the paramedics arrive, they ask Mom to walk the hallway. She says, "My knee hurts a little, but I think I'm okay." They assess her injuries as non-critical and, together, we agree she doesn't need an ambulance ride. They recommend a follow-up with her doctor if the pain worsens.

But within the hour, doubt creeps in. Mom, the caregiver, and I all second-guess our decision. *Maybe she should be evaluated more thoroughly?* What follows is a stressful scramble—my sister and the caregiver helping Mom into the car with a possible knee fracture, hours spent in the ER waiting room, and a battle to convince staff she needs to be admitted.

Looking back, the better path was clear: let the fall speak for itself. An eighty-three-year-old woman living alone, reporting pain and possible broken bones, arriving by ambulance would have triggered a more immediate and appropriate response upon arriving at the ER. Follow your instincts.

A lesson learned is that if you call 911, follow through with having the paramedics transport the elder to the hospital. Chances are that even after a first responder evaluation, the elder may still need a more thorough examination, and paramedics have the skills and equipment needed to lift and transport your loved one safely. Don't second-guess yourself. Send the patient to the hospital; the ambulance is ready and waiting.

Hospital Admission, Again

At the hospital, Mom goes through the usual drill—bloodwork, x-rays, and a head-to-toe assessment. The good news is that nothing is broken this time, but she has knee pain and skin abrasions.

The tests also reveal a urinary tract infection and some concerning lab results, enough to warrant admission. And just like that, we're back in a rinse and repeat hospital-to-rehab cycle along with a 'fresh' new set of orders for physical and occupational therapy to reduce the risk of future falls.

After a few days, Mom is discharged to a rehab facility. I've learned my lesson, and this time I approach things differently. We're more proactive, communicating regularly with the care team, social worker, physician and nurses, and reinforcing the reality that Mom lives alone, I live out of state, and she must regain enough strength to manage safely on her own.

Instead of rushing the process or pushing for her release simply because a respite arrangement is already in place, we focus on maximizing the rehab services. If there is medical justification, Mom can remain in rehab beyond standard Medicare coverage because her supplemental insurance can continue paying once Medicare drops off, provided the services are deemed medically necessary. Let the process and her recovery play out organically, rather than moving her too quickly just because the next place has space available.

Research and understand what insurance coverage applies to rehab facility services and if there is supplemental insurance, learn how these resources can subsidize Medicare coverage.

"While You Recover"- Temporary Words, a Permanent Stay

As Mom wraps up her rehab stay, we can now transition her to an assisted living facility. We explain to her that, just like last time, she's not quite ready to return home, and she needs another "stop-off at respite care," the same assisted living facility where she's previously stayed. The part we leave out is that this time, instead of being a respite, short-term stay, we are renting a one-bedroom apartment and moving her into the assisted living facility permanently.

THE RUSE—MOM'S 'NOT SO TEMPORARY' STAY AT ASSISTED LIVING

Since Mom previously stayed at this assisted living facility for respite care, and since we have a relationship with the staff, all are onboard participating in our ruse. We are telling Mom she's staying here 'while' she recovers, but the truth is, this is a permanent move. We all agree to use phrases like, *while you recover* and *as you get stronger* as she settles in.

The hope is that she'll acclimate before we are forced to come clean, and we can avoid a full-on fight. She will hate it when we tell her the truth, but change is needed, and she is already out of her house. This is the perfect time to make the move.

We are ready for take-off. The staff is aligned, and our covert plan is set in motion. Now we must execute. There is a lot to do to get Mom's assisted living apartment set up before she arrives. It's Wednesday, and she is being released from rehab on Monday.

Mom's new home is a one-bedroom, one-bath with a living space and a kitchenette. It's a nice space that needs furnishing before she arrives. If we could include Mom in this process, we'd discuss what furniture she'd like moved from home. But collaborating with her isn't an option. We can't have her enter this new place, *where she's supposedly staying for respite care,* and see all her personal belongings. Mom is smart, so we need to outsmart her. We devise a plan, set a budget, and kick off our shopping spree, starting with a local discount furniture store.

We power shop for a sofa, end tables, a television stand, and a small kitchen table. We splurge on a big TV since Mom's daylong social companions are the cast of Hallmark movies. She deserves a new television, and she will never buy it for herself. She always worries about running out of money.

Tina donates a spare twin bed, and we spruce it up with a new headboard. We raid Mom's basement. Dust off a few lamps, a large mirror and an old microwave cart I threw out years ago. Mom couldn't see it going to waste, so she rescued it from the curb before the garbage truck arrived. Dad rolled his eyes as she loaded it into their van and hauled it back to St. Louis following a visit to Texas. We resurrect Mom's 'treasure' as a barista bar housing her decades-old Mr. Coffee.

Late Sunday night, Tina and I wrap up the finishing touches. All the furniture is assembled, and the shower curtain is hung. The pantry is stocked with Mom's favorite snacks, and a welcome wreath hangs on the door. *Our work here is done.* Mom's new home is perfect and ready for her arrival.

It is Monday morning. The rehab center and assisted living facility coordinate transportation, and I watch as Mom is wheeled into the accessible van. Once inside, her wheelchair is locked in place. I am giddy with anticipation, hoping she'll love her new place, even if she *thinks* it is only for respite care.

Arriving at the assisted living facility, the staff greets her with love and enthusiasm. Her disposition is pleasant, but cautious. She'd rather be going home. We make our way to her apartment, and she comments on the door wreath. This is a good start. We enter, and she looks around. "This is very nice. It looks a lot different from when I was here before," she says.

"Isn't it homey?" I say, shifting her focus.

"Oh yes," she says. "It reminds me a lot of my house. I have lamps just like those."

Mission accomplished, at least for now. We've created Mom's new home with just enough of her own things to feel familiar. And we've avoided a major confrontation of telling her she's never returning to her home. She lives here now.

We spend much of the day getting her settled, coordinating with the nurse about her medications, and ensuring she has an escort to the dining hall because she's claustrophobic and won't ride the elevator from the second to the first floor by herself.

As the day draws to a close, I return to Mom's house where I am staying, flop into bed, exhale and stare at the ceiling. A tear rolls down my cheek. *Success. We did it.* She's settled in at her new place. She's happy, or at least as happy as we can expect, and she'll be safe there.

Day 2 at Her New Place

The next day I work a little while at the house, but I'm distracted. *I hope Mom had a good night's rest. I wonder how she is doing?* By lunchtime, I log off and head over to check in on her. I enter her apartment to find her in her wheelchair at the kitchen table with a half-eaten grilled cheese in a Styrofoam container in front of her. I kiss her on the head and ask, "How are you doing? How'd you sleep?"

Mom is in a foul mood. I'm annoyed. When I left yesterday, everything was good, or at least I convinced myself it was. She is in her new place, and my 'project milestones' are marked complete. She now just needs to settle in. But it's clear that's not happening. Today, she's argumentative. Primed for a fight about anything.

Doesn't she know how hard I've worked to set up her new home? Of course she doesn't. She can't because we can't tell her. Last night's feeling of success is erased by a single scowl on Mom's face. *I may never outgrow my desire for her approval.*

"What's wrong?" I ask.

"Room service just brought my lunch. I didn't even get breakfast," she says. "And I didn't sleep at all last night. That bed is too small." I dismiss the comment about room service and focus on her sleeping. I reassure her that the twin bed is the same size as the one she slept in at rehab for four weeks. "No. That was a full-size bed," she insists. Instead of fighting her, I leverage her obstinacy against her.

"Mom, this is the furniture provided," I say, "If you think you'll sleep better, how about I bring your bed from home?"

"That would be great," she says, "But I don't want you to go to any trouble."

Bam. Another win. She just agreed to allow me to move her bed from home to the assisted living apartment. I'm ecstatic. "It is no trouble at all. I'll load it in the van, and the facility manager can help me set it up." *Unbelievable. Everything is falling into place except for that one comment about room service,* but I choose to ignore it. For the moment, I'm feeling too good. *Maybe she's accepting this transition more easily than I thought she would?*

I hurry back to Mom's house. With sweat dripping from every part of me, I singlehandedly wrestle the fullsize mattress and bedframe into the minivan and race back to the assisted living center, hoping to get some help unloading and setting up the bed before the maintenance supervisor clocks out for the day. *I can't believe it.* Mom is settled in her new home. Her clothes are in the drawers, her plants are on the window ledge, her *barista* bar is stocked, her beer is in the refrigerator, and her tub of pretzels is on the kitchen table. My work here is done, for now. I know there will be more challenges, but I don't want to think about them right now. Mom's resistance to change means her temporary satisfaction with her bed from home will be short-lived. She's destined to complain about something else, but for now, I'll take the win. Tina and I have done a great job, and I opt to relish the joy. I'm excited to be heading home.

The next morning before dawn I board the plane and settle into my familiar row-eight seat. I exhale and reflect on all that has happened. Mom's health is declining. She is getting older. She can't take care of herself anymore and she's never returning home.

With the whirlwind of events behind me, emotion sets in. *What have I done? I did what needs to be done. Mom needs help. She needs to be safe. Tina and I can't keep supporting her in her home. It is taking a toll on our health. This is the right decision. Isn't it? I love her, and I want what is best for her, but I just uprooted her from her home, and she doesn't even know it.*

> *Each elder care situation is unique. Some circumstances are constrained by finances, others by strained relationships, and others by cognitive decline brought on by dementia or Alzheimer's. Whatever decisions you and the care team make, if they align with providing the best health and safety for the elder balanced alongside the mental, emotional and physical wellbeing of the family care team, it is the right decision.*

I land in Texas. My husband picks me up from the airport, and I unwind at home, unpack my suitcase, kiss the dog, and hug my husband. Despite the two-hour flight, flipping roles from caregiver to Mom to wife and mother doesn't happen instantly. My husband notices that I'm distracted. I'm back home, but I'm not present. My thoughts are still with Mom in St. Louis.

"Are you okay?" he asks. "How's your mom doing?"

"She's getting old. I'm sad for her," I say. "I'm not sure how much longer she'll be with us." Our dialogue drifts off. I open the airline app on my phone and search for flights. *I need to get Rick and the kids to St. Louis to visit Mom before she dies.*

Two Truths: Her Decline, My Quiet Aching

A few weeks pass. I settle back into my life in Texas just in time to hop on a plane and head back to St. Louis. I'm thankful this time that it isn't a crisis visit where I'm scrambling to find the next flight out. Instead, this visit is planned with Rick and the kids; Adam, Meagan (Adam's fiancée), and Parker joining me. I'm excited to show off Mom's new apartment, and since Meagan has never met her, I'm sure this will be the perfect visit. *Forgotten lesson number one: lower my expectations.*

On the way to the assisted living center, we stop at a convenience store to buy lottery scratch-offs. When Adam was in college, he'd visit Mardy (my mom), and they'd sit at her kitchen table, drink a beer and scratch off tickets together. He wants to introduce his wife-to-be and share this fond memory.

Before going directly to Mom's apartment, I take my crew on a quick tour of the facility, showing off the movie theater with the popcorn cart parked near the entrance. We visit the lounge where the residents gather for happy hour, and we pass by the dining room where the staff is setting up for a singalong with Sam, a local musician who plays favorite tunes, everything from Elvis' *Blue Suede Shoes* to Jim Croce's *Bad Bad Leroy Brown*.

Residents gather with smiles, singing and clapping as Sam fills the room with familiar melodies from decades past. A few roll onto the dance floor, swaying in rhythm with wheelchairs and walkers. As the tour winds down, I point out the activities calendar posted near the elevators. Field trips, a gardening club, ice cream socials, and community service events are all part of the lineup, offering connection, purpose, and a bit of fun.

We make our way to Mom's apartment. She's expecting me, but not my husband and the kids. *Mistake number two: Don't surprise Mom. It rarely goes well.* I'm the first one through the door. A foul odor slaps me in the face. *Good Lord, what is that?*

"Hi Mom. I'm here. Look who I brought with me," I announce. She's still in bed. It's three in the afternoon. "How are you feeling?" I ask. I assess the situation and quickly realize the stench I'm smelling is coming from her. She is unkempt and looks as if she's not brushed her teeth or showered for days.

She stinks, and I'm feeling sick. I'm embarrassed, humiliated and upset. *I bring my family all the way here from Texas, and you can't even get a shower, brush your hair and put on clean clothes?*

Taking inventory, I notice food crumbs and portions of meals litter the floor in the kitchenette, and on the counter sits a stack of empty Styrofoam containers. I open the refrigerator and discover a can of soda lying on its side, with its contents dripping onto the shelves below.

What's going on? I was here a few weeks ago, and the place looked perfect. This isn't like Mom. I've been calling her every few days and exchanging emails with the director of nursing, who said that she is struggling to adjust, but overall, she is doing well. *Not from what I can tell.*

I step into the hall and head to the nurses' station. I need an update from the nurse's aide. She says that they have been encouraging Mom to engage, but she refuses. She declines help with showering. "Someone has to be in the apartment with her while she bathes, and she doesn't like that," the care partner explains.

"So, she's not bathing. We encourage her, but we can't force her. She's very strong-willed." *She sure is. And I need you to be more resilient. You need to make her shower.* My feelings of embarrassment and frustration now transform into anger and resentment. *How could she do this? She's not even trying.*

"What's with all the empty containers in her room?" I ask. "And her kitchen floor is a mess," I say.

"She refuses to go to the dining hall. She says she wants to eat in her room." She thinks she's in a hotel. In hindsight, maybe I should have taken her comment about calling down for "room service" more seriously. *She's not buying in. She's not acclimating.* Although familiar faces surround her, residents she met during a previous stay, she refuses to engage. They invite her to join them for meals and activities, but she declines.

As I continue probing the staff and matching the series of events against Mom's version, my emotions flip-flop. *Maybe I shouldn't be mad at her. Maybe I should pity her.*

It turns out she gave the dining hall a try when she first arrived. But the experience left her shaken. "I made a mess. I can't even feed myself," she said, before breaking down in tears.

"I got ready for breakfast one morning. I let the girl help me. I went down to the dining hall. I even rode in the elevator. The girl talked to me the whole time, so I wasn't scared. She wheeled me up to a table with people I didn't know, and I tried making conversation with them. When I reached for my orange juice, the glass slipped out of my hands, and I spilled it all down my shirt and into my lap. I was so embarrassed. These damn hands don't work. I can't hold onto anything."

Her neuropathy is progressing, and as much as I want to stay mad at her, I can't. She's in pain—mental, physical and emotional. She's slipping. Losing her ability to take care of her basic needs, like bathing and eating. Now I'm crying.

Her time here is limited; that much is clear, and the weight of that truth is hard to carry. Her needs are evolving quickly, outpacing what assisted living can reasonably provide. In just a few months, another move will be necessary. A higher level of care is no longer a distant probability; it's becoming an urgent reality.

CHAPTER 15

When Assisted Living Isn't Enough—The Move to Long-Term Care

Topics

- Mom's Being Kicked Out—Bless Her Heart

- When "Settled" Isn't Permanent: Navigating Yet Another Move with Mom

- Making It Feel Like Home—Even When Downsizing Again

- Tech with Heart: Adapting to Neuropathy with Smart Solutions

- The Old Phone Number—My Lifeline

- Gentle Openers: Talking with a Parent Who's Feeling Low

Getting Mom settled into her assisted living apartment is a major milestone, one more box checked on the ever-growing project plan. We transformed a modest one-bedroom apartment into a warm, familiar space, layering in the comforts of home. And she hates it.

She wants to live out the rest of her life in her three-bedroom ranch home just a few miles away. But this is what she needs now. She has care staff for managing meds and bathing. She has nutritious meals, activities, amenities, and instant companionship. Still, she isn't adjusting and the aggressive neuropathy, resulting from a neck injury, is taking over her body. Despite receiving physical therapy twice a week, her strength continues to fade. She can no longer maneuver a walker safely and now relies entirely on a wheelchair. Feeding herself has become a struggle; more often than not, the food lands in her lap instead of her mouth.

And even as I watch Mom's rapid decline, I deny that her needs are outpacing what this facility can offer. In my mind, *she's okay for now.* She's safe. She's being cared for. And so, with a naïve sense of security, my husband and I head off to Mexico over Labor Day weekend.

Mom's Being Kicked Out of Assisted Living— Bless Her Heart

When we land, I switch off airplane mode, and my phone lights up with a flood of texts from my sister. *Check your email. It's about Mom. There's a message from Joanne—the assisted living director.*

So much for a quiet weekend. My shoulders tense as I'm pulled back into problem-solving mode. *Should I catch the next flight to St. Louis?*

Joanne's email is direct:

"…your mother's care needs are progressing and require a level of service we cannot provide. She's becoming fully lift-dependent, meaning she cannot support her own weight. She needs two care team members to transfer her to and from her wheelchair. You will need to make different arrangements for her over the next few weeks."

Did Joanne really need to send this on the Friday before a holiday weekend? Emotions bounce from fear: *What do we do next? Where does she go from here?* To: *This isn't a crisis we need to handle in the next two days. I don't have to catch the next flight out.*

I write back:

"Joanne, thank you for letting us know. I'm sure this isn't the outcome you hope for any of your residents. We wish she could stay, but we understand. I'm asking—pleading—for your help in giving us time to research and find a new place that can meet her needs. Can she stay there for the next few weeks while we make arrangements?"

We exchange a few more messages. Joanne reassures me, Mom won't be discharged until we find her a new place. Immediate crisis averted.

Still, her follow-up stings.

"We want what's best for her, but she's a handful. She is a lot to deal with between her physical needs and temperamental behavior."

Within a few short months of moving into assisted living, Mom is being kicked out in the nicest way possible. The van's backseat is still a garden of fake Ficus leaves and Mom's on the move again. It feels like a bad rerun of Groundhog Day only with aging parent care.

Studies show that on average older adults now spend about a year in assisted living, down from nearly two years not long ago. This decline is due to a variety of reasons, the most significant being that older adults are entering assisted living later, often with more advanced health conditions such as dementia, high blood pressure, and heart disease. This means their health is already in a state of more rapid decline when they move in, shortening the time until they need a higher level of care. Additionally, in-home care options have expanded, and the rising cost of assisted living makes families delay the move as long as possible.

> Housing and healthcare costs associated with aging are continuously increasing. Per a U.S. News report released in the summer of 2024 citing 2023 data from Genworth Financial, the average monthly cost for a nursing home ranges between $8,669 for a semi-private room and $9,733 for a private room.
>
> Most nursing home residents in the United States—over 60 percent—depend on Medicaid to pay for their long-term care, according to the American Health Care Association.
>
> A fundamental difference between Medicare and Medicaid is that Medicare is a federal health insurance program mainly for people sixty-five and older, while Medicaid is a state and federal assistance program that provides health coverage for people with low income and limited resources.

When "Settled" Isn't Permanent: Navigating Yet Another Move with Mom

My critical thinking and research skills kick back in as I hunt for Mom's next accommodations, a long-term care facility. Leveraging lessons from the last go-round, I've refined my search. I have only two leads to follow. One is already on my radar from earlier rounds of researching assisted-living facilities (many senior living campuses offer tiered care options ranging from independent living to assisted living, with step ups to long-term or memory care). The other is a personal referral, a friend's father-in-law lived there, and the family spoke highly of the care he received.

The one facility already on my radar requires financial transparency. They want to know that Mom has at least three years of financial liquidity before considering her. Initially, I am offended, but after learning that the average life expectancy for a nursing home resident is three years, the request seems more logical.

It is heartbreaking for an elder who acclimates to a community, makes friends and makes it their home to be uprooted because they run out of money. Moving a loved one when they are most vulnerable is difficult for everyone—the elder, their new friends, the family and the nursing home care team. So, knowing that the future occupant has enough money to stay at the facility through the duration of their life makes sense.

We visit the second option on my list, the personal recommendation, and fall in love with it. This facility is set up like a neighborhood with standalone houses, each having a maximum of ten residents and a ratio of ten elders for every two care partners, plus a nurse.

Each cottage mate has their own bedroom and bathroom, and the environment is homey. Entering through the front door feels like walking into a family home with a large, central kitchen and adjoining living room featuring a big TV and fireplace. I know right away. *This is it. This is Mom's next home.*

GETTING MOM'S BUY-IN FOR ANOTHER MOVE

Explaining to Mom that she's on the move again isn't easy, and my emotions are bouncing somewhere between angry and sad. Part of me believes she sabotaged the assisted living arrangement, refusing to engage, resisting every effort to help. But another part of me understands it's not her fault. Her body is simply failing her. I know the decline isn't something she is choosing.

Mom refuses to accept the assisted living facility. She complains constantly about the staff, the food, and the routines. So, I use her frustration as leverage when broaching the subject of moving *again*. I build up the new place, show her pictures, and describe the welcoming, homelike environment. She's not buying it.

She wants to go back home. She wants her caregivers back. But that's impractical. She needs round-the-clock care, and that staying in her home is cost-prohibitive and unmanageable. The revolving door of caregivers, the risk of her being alone—it's too much for me and Tina to manage. She's unable to move without the assistance of two people! She needs a nursing home, but I can't tell her this. She'll resist, fight and make the transition harder than it needs to be. I don't have it in me to go there.

I shift my angle. My strategy is to frame the new place as a better version of the facility where she is staying now. Since she doesn't fully grasp the distinctions between independent living, assisted living, and long-term care, I hope she doesn't notice the differences right away. Eventually, we'll need to address the financial implications, but for now, the priority is getting her moved.

Making It Feel Like Home—Even When Downsizing Again

With each relocation, Mom's world shrinks a little more. What once filled a four-bedroom, three-bath home has been pared down to fit inside a modest two-room assisted living apartment. Now, transitioning to long-term care, even fewer belongings come with her.

Despite the cozy, inviting common areas, the individual rooms are a bit sparse. Her personal space consists of a vinyl recliner—heavy and clinical, parked in the corner—and a wooden dresser that doubles as a TV stand. The comforts of home have been whittled down to what's functional, what fits, what's allowed.

Instead of a linen closet, she has three open shelves tucked into the bathroom wall. The shower and toilet share one continuous space, no divider, just a gently sloped floor with a central drain to catch runoff from sponge baths or the inevitable accidents that come with aging bodies.

We stock the dresser drawers with a handful of t-shirts and sweatpants. A minimal wardrobe is all that's needed here.

To soften the sterile feel, we bring in her plant stands and dress them with familiar greenery: the Christmas cactus, the African violet, the fern. She can't water them on her own anymore; the care team helps with that, but she still talks to them. They're living company, longtime friends.

Outside her window, we hang a bird feeder from a shepherd's hook. Mom loves nature, and the sight of a cardinal pecking at seeds brings a flicker of joy to her face. These small touches—plants, birds, color—are our way of keeping her world alive.

We place a digital picture frame on a small table near her bed, uploading fresh images every so often—snapshots of her grandkids, blooming flowers, and beloved dogs. I also print a few dozen 4x6 photos, frame them, and mount them on the wall just inside her doorway. The blank space becomes a gallery of familiar faces and memories, a natural conversation starter and something she and anyone who visits can enjoy.

Another place we add a personal touch is the shadow box outside her room. Each resident has one—a narrow box for a name card and a few photos. We keep Mom's box festive, swapping out the background with seasonal scenes: a yellow felt square with tiny lights and garden gnomes for spring, shamrocks and a pot of gold for St. Patrick's Day, jack-o'-lanterns for Halloween, and ornaments and a tree for Christmas. Personalizing her room makes it a little homier.

I know she notices. I know it matters. But sometimes I wonder if I do it more for her or for me.

Tech with Heart: Adapting to Neuropathy with Smart Solutions

Along with the digital picture frame, we've outfitted Mom's room with adaptive technology to support her worsening neuropathy, which increasingly limits the use of her hands. Her table lamp is now connected to a smart outlet, allowing her to control it with simple voice commands: "Alexa, turn the lamp on in the bedroom," or "Alexa, turn the lamp off." It's a brilliant solution when it works.

The real challenge is twofold: helping her remember how to use it and making sure the staff doesn't unplug it and accidentally reset the programming. The first requires ongoing reminders and coaching. She mumbles through the commands or says light instead of lamp, confusing Alexa. The second challenge is managed with a bold "Do Not Unplug" sign taped above the outlet.

We've also synced her TV to respond to voice commands. Saying "Alexa, turn on the TV" brings the screen to life, and she can adjust the volume or change channels without fumbling for buttons. These innovations extend her independence, giving her a bit more control in a world that's growing increasingly limited.

THE GARDEN CLUB

Mom shares her cottage house with nine other women, each with her own story—woven with many common threads. They bond over the St. Louis Cardinals and the rhythm of local news, and they all share a love for plants. Come spring, they take pride in tending the courtyard, keeping the perennials healthy and blooming.

One staff member even builds a raised flower box from reclaimed wood. It stands on stilts, perfectly positioned at wheelchair height so the residents can dig, water, and nurture the soil with ease. One side is reserved for flowers; the other, for vegetables—cucumbers and tomatoes that they watch grow with pride and satisfaction. What happens here is more than gardening. It's connection, purpose, and a little bit of joy rooted in the earth.

One unexpected benefit that comes from Mom living in long-term care is that she's no longer alone at mealtimes. Unlike her previous assisted living setup where she often opted for 'room service' and solitude, this facility encourages communal dining. Staff help her get up, dressed, and wheeled into the dining room, where she's surrounded by other residents.

She grumbles, of course. *"I hate that they make me eat three meals a day. I eat slow, and my stomach's not that big."* But we're relieved. She's getting balanced meals, and she's in a space that nudges her toward connection. It takes time, but eventually she begins to acclimate, sharing small talk, trading glances, and slowly building rapport with her housemates. The dining room becomes more than a place to eat; it's an invitation to belong.

Dietitians and culinary staff work to ensure that menus are not only enjoyable but also meet the unique nutritional needs of seniors, such as promoting good hydration, strong bone density, and muscle mass. This includes incorporating essential components like lean proteins, whole grains, healthy fats, and fiber-rich foods.

The Old Phone Number—My Lifeline

I'm grateful Mom is socializing. It's good for her to be out of her room, connecting with the other cottage mates. But ironically, because she's not in her room as much, it's harder for me to reach her by phone. Living out of state means I can't swing by after work or drop in on a Sunday afternoon. So, I rely on phone calls to stay connected.

When Mom was still at home and even when she moved into assisted living, I could call her. Her legacy landline number followed her wherever she lived, until now. Sometimes, when she didn't answer right away, I'd leave a message on her answering machine, rambling on just long enough for her to safely make her way to the phone and pick up. Since she's relocated to the nursing home, our conversations are less frequent. Despite my best efforts to stay engaged, the line is cut, disconnected.

Mom and Dad's old phone number was more than just a string of digits. It was a connection to their past. Neighbors, high school friends, Dad's golf buddies, former colleagues, they all knew Mom and Dad's number. Most of my parents' generation don't connect through texts or social media. Instead, they keep up with each other through phone calls and obituary notices. And now that communication link is broken, metaphorically and physically.

With Mom's latest relocation to the nursing home, not only is she having to adjust to change, but I am, too. I now have to dial the facility's main phone number to reach her, a logistical hurdle for me and the staff. The social worker offers a solution: schedule a standing call each week so they can make sure Mom is in her room, ready to talk.

This sounds good, but it doesn't work for me. I've got to rev myself up to talk with her; emotional prep is half the battle. Knowing every Tuesday at 8 p.m. I'm calling Mom, I'd start dreading Tuesdays more than Mondays.

I can't commit to that. I need flexibility to be able to call when I've got the bandwidth, when the day hasn't drained me, when I've exercised and I can pivot the conversation away from complaints with updates about the kids.

Sometimes I wait for a text from Tina: *"Mom's in a pretty good mood today if you want to call."* That's my cue to connect.

Today, it's one of the good days. Work went smoothly, my mind feels clear, and I've got the emotional fortitude to talk to her. I scroll through my contacts, locate the nursing home and tap call. Two rings and the connection is made–the adventure begins.

"Press one to reach a staff member. Press two to reach an elder staying with us."

The automated voice continues: "Press one for House One, press two for House Two…" I tap four.

"Please hold while your call is being transferred."

I wait. The ringing begins. I lean my head back, close my eyes, and start counting. Sometimes I make it to twenty. Other times, I give up around fifteen and press end. *I'll try again tomorrow*—partly relieved, partly disappointed. I had hoped to check the "Call Mom" item off my to-do list today, but since we don't connect, the task rolls forward.

The other version of this ritual, the 'lucky one,' is when a care partner picks up. When this happens, the scenario plays out something like this…

"Hi. This is Marlene's daughter, Kathy. Is Marlene at the table or in the living area, or is she in her room?"

"Who?"

"Marlene. This is her daughter."

"Oh. We have two Marlenes. Which did you want to talk to?"

"Marlene in room four, please," I struggle to remain pleasant.

"Oh. I think she's at the table. Sorry. I'm covering for one of the care partners tonight. I don't usually work in this building. I don't know all their names yet."

"It's okay. I appreciate you picking up. Do you think you could get her on the phone?"

"Well. I answered the phone in the office. This isn't the cordless phone. So, I don't have a way of getting it to her. Do you think you could call back? I'll answer on the cordless next time."

"Sure," turning the phone speaker away from my mouth so she can't hear me sigh. "I'll call right back."

We disconnect. I press redial and once again navigate the phone prompts. The ringing starts. One, two, three...

"Hello. This is Teresa."

Only three rings this time. Progress.

"Hi Teresa. This is Kathy again. Marlene's daughter. Did you answer on the cordless?"

"I sure did, and I'm standing right next to her." Her voice becomes more distant as I hear Teresa say, "Here you go Ms. Marlene. It's your daughter."

I hear Mom say, "Oh. Honey, I can't hold it. I'll drop it." *Clank. Swish. Scuffle.* The two of them wrestle to rescue the phone that I visualize has slithered somewhere between Mom's leg and the arm of the wheelchair.

"Here. I got it." I hear Teresa say.

I scream into my phone. "Teresa! Teresa! Can you hear me? She needs you to put it on speaker."

"Honey. Can you put it on speakerphone?" Mom asks.

"I don't know how to do that," I hear Teresa's voice off in the distance.

I scream again, "Teresa! Can you hear me? Teresa, talk to me. It's the green button."

"Hello ma'am," Teresa's voice is clearer. She's regained control of the phone. She begins, "I don't..."

I interrupt. "Press the green talk button. It's the same button you use to answer the cordless phone. Pressing it again puts it on speaker."

She presses the talk button. "Can you hear us?"

"Yes, I can."

"Hooray. You did it. Great job, honey," Mom says.

Every single time. Every time I call, it's the same thing. None of the care partners knows how to put the phone on speaker. *How do I know?* I asked. Last time I visited I asked the care partner on duty how to do it. Unfortunately, she's no longer there. With the phone now on speaker and finally propped on the table in front of Mom, our conversation begins.

"Hi honey. I'm glad you called. It's great to hear your voice," she begins, crying.

"Hi Mom. I'm glad to hear your voice, too. I've been thinking about you."

More crying. "I've been down. I'm depressed. I have nothing to say." More crying.

I start in with an event of the day. "So, let me tell you about Adam and Meagan…"

Calling is a hassle on so many levels, before, during, and after I make contact with her.

Gentle Openers: Talking with a Parent Who's Feeling Low

When an aging parent is feeling low, connection can be fragile. The goal isn't to force cheerfulness, but to gently invite engagement, spark memory, or offer comfort.

> Here are some conversation starters that balance warmth, curiosity, and emotional safety:
>
> - **"What was your favorite season growing up?"** Let her talk about the weather, holidays, or childhood routines. Nostalgia can be grounding.
>
> - **"Tell me about a neighbor you really liked."** This can open the door to stories about community, friendship, or even gossip.
>
> - **"Do you remember when [grandchild's name] was little and did that funny thing?"** Shared memories build emotional bridges and remind her of her legacy.

- **"I saw a dog today that looked just like [former pet's name]. It made me think of you."** Animal memories often bring warmth and comfort.

- **"If you could have any dessert tonight, what would it be?"** Food is a safe and often joyful topic.

- **"What song always made you want to dance?"** Music can unlock emotion and memory, even in moments of depression.

RESOURCES

What Is the Average Length of Stay in Assisted Living? (seniorservicesofamerica.com).

Adaptive Technology

Nursing Home Dietary—Nutrition

Family connectedness—phone calls, drop ins

CHAPTER 16

Crazy Stuff Happens with a UTI

Topics

— Understanding UTIs: What Are They and the Symptoms You Might Not Expect

— Seeing What isn't There: Responding to Hallucinations with Compassion

— PureWick Explained: A Non-Invasive Catheter Option

— Rehab Services in Long-Term Care: What to Expect When Living There Permanently

— Getting Home from the Hospital: The Private Ambulance Option

When Mom gets urinary tract infections (UTIs), the lesson for the care team member is this: if she is talking crazy, don't assume she's ready for memory care—it just might hurt to pee. When did swapping kid stories about academic achievements or big game wins turn into trying to one-up friends with stories about the crazy stuff Mom did when she had a UTI? And the stories? They're wild. UTIs in older adults can trigger bizarre, erratic behaviors that catch families, and even medical professionals, off guard.

It's important to understand how common this is. Unlike younger patients, elders often don't show the usual signs like cloudy urine or burning during urination. Instead, elder-onset UTIs can masquerade as cognitive decline, presenting as confusion, agitation, hallucinations, loss of coordination, and sudden falls. It's no wonder families and clinicians sometimes mistake these symptoms for dementia or Alzheimer's. When a UTI causes hallucinations, it's terrifying—for the elder and for those who love them. The disorientation is real, and the emotional toll is heavy.

Understanding UTIs: What They Are and the Symptoms You Might Not Expect

Mom's first, "*She did what*?" moment happened one New Year's Eve Day. My husband and I had traveled to Mexico for the holiday when I got a call from my sister. This is how the conversation unfolded.

"Kath, we just got to Mom's house. Something is off," Tina said. "All the lights are on. The kitchen cabinets are wide open. There's food on the counter and a Rubbermaid lid she used as a bowl, filled with Cheerios and milk."

She explained that Mom was still in bed. When Tina asked her about the mess, Mom calmly explained she'd been feeding the dogs and cats.

Mom doesn't have pets.

"She sounded perfectly normal when I talked to her on the phone yesterday. Now she's acting erratic and confused," Tina said.

Was this the beginning of Alzheimer's? Should we start looking into memory care?

We talked through the incident and decided that whatever was going on, it could wait until after the holiday. Then, Tina said, "I wonder if Mom has a UTI?"

"Maybe," I responded. "But what does that have to do with her being delusional?"

Turns out, everything.

Urinary tract infections are common in older adults—especially women—and they don't always show up the way we'd expect. Forget the classic symptoms like burning or pain during urination. Elders may not feel these sensations at all, or they may not be able to articulate them.

Instead, UTIs in aging adults often manifest as confusion, agitation, or bizarre behavior. Why? Because the bladder stays full too long. Whether it's the third trip to the bathroom in the middle of the night that feels like too much effort, or the reluctance to ask for help in a facility, elders often hold it. That stagnant urine becomes a breeding ground for bacteria, and a UTI is born.

It's not memory loss. It's not dementia. It's biology. And it's one of the most misunderstood triggers of sudden cognitive changes in older adults.

No two UTI stories are alike, but their characteristics have eerie similarities. The first time a UTI triggers odd behavior in an aging parent, it is unsettling. But the longer I serve as the project manager of Mom's life, when she's not herself, my first thought isn't dementia or decline. It's: Could this be a UTI?

A urinary tract infection is an infection in any part of the urinary system. The urinary system includes kidneys, ureters, bladder and urethra. To determine if a UTI is present, a urine sample is taken and cultured to determine the specific bacteria present. For specifics on UTIs, check out the Mayo Clinic webpage Urinary tract infection (UTI) - Symptoms and causes.

Depending on the type of bacteria, specific antibiotics are prescribed. The tricky part is knowing whether they're actually working. *How can we tell if Mom is no longer infected?*

When we ask the medical team to retest her ten to fourteen days after starting treatment, we're met with resistance. "That's not common practice. It takes time for the medication to work. And with older adults, it's nearly impossible to get a clean catch. There are always some bacteria in the urine."

Common practice or not, it's frustrating. If we never confirm whether the infection has cleared, how do we know if Mom's behavior is the lingering result of a UTI or something more serious?

The simple, unsatisfying answer: we don't. And that uncertainty leaves caregivers stuck in a loop of guesswork, hoping we're treating the right problem.

UTI Delirium

UTI delirium refers to a state of sudden confusion and altered mental status that can occur in older adults because of a urinary tract infection (UTI). Both the infection and the body's immune response to it can lead to changes in brain function, causing symptoms like disorientation, hallucinations, and memory problems. Some may also present with symptoms of aggression, withdrawal, and restlessness.

HOW IS A UTI DIAGNOSED IN A PERSON WITH DELIRIUM?

Making a UTI diagnosis in a person with delirium is not always straightforward. As already mentioned, delirium may be the only noticeable symptom of a UTI in older adults. This is because it's hard to tell if adults who are bedbound or have dementia are having pain when urinating or having to urinate more often. They also may be unable to communicate their symptoms. Or if they wear diapers for incontinence (not being able to control their bladder or bowel function), it's hard to tell how often they urinate.

HOW DOES A UTI AFFECT THE BRAIN?

I don't understand how a urinary tract infection (UTI) affects the brain, and it seems medical professionals are also asking the same question. While scientists haven't pinpointed the exact connection between UTIs and delirium, they have some ideas. When we get an infection, our immune system jumps into action, releasing chemicals that cause inflammation. These chemicals often contribute to symptoms like fatigue and fever. In older adults, the brain is more susceptible to this inflammation and the stress hormones the body produces to fight the infection. This inflammation and stress on the brain may manifest as delirium.

So, why don't young, healthy adults typically get delirium from infections like UTIs? It comes down to the blood-brain barrier, a special shield between the brain and the rest of the body. This barrier keeps harmful bacteria, viruses, and fungi from reaching the brain. In older adults, this barrier isn't as robust, making their brains more vulnerable to the inflammation caused by infections, according to "Can UTIs Cause Confusion?—GoodRx."

Seeing What isn't There: Responding to Hallucinations with Compassion

Mom's wacky behavior of feeding invisible dogs and cats in her kitchen was the first of many UTIs. While at the nursing home, she is diagnosed with chronic UTIs, with one that earned her a first-class ambulance ride to the hospital, and me a boomerang trip back to St. Louis.

I pack for a quick three-day trip, hoping to be home with my immediate family by Saturday so we can celebrate the Easter weekend together. I should know better. That doesn't happen.

Despite the high dose, intravenous antibiotics for three days, her doctor isn't comfortable discharging her on Friday. She will be 'celebrating' Easter in the hospital.

Mid-morning on Holy Saturday, I enter Mom's hospital room with a bouquet of artificial Texas bluebonnets, a vase and twinkle lights. Mom smiles. We exchange niceties. She tells me she's been getting Tylenol every four hours for neck pain, and she recently had a dose of Gabapentin. Mom's C3/C4 neck fracture causes her chronic discomfort. Often, she powers through it, but sometimes it is debilitating. The neuropathy extending from her hands, through her extremities, and up her spine, coupled with anxiety and any brain misfiring brought on by the UTI, leaves her feeling as if she wants to crawl out of her skin. And with a bit too much Gabapentin for pain, hallucinations rise to a whole new level.

RANDOM ACT OF KINDNESS

I notice that nestled next to Mom's hip is a plush gray teddy bear. "He's cute. Where did you get him?" I ask.

"The lady across the hall gave him to me," she says.

That doesn't sound right. She has no relationship with the patient across the hall. I dismiss her answer, assuming she's confused.

A few minutes later, the nurse steps into the room. Speaking in code so as not to alarm Mom, she gives me an update: Mom is struggling. She is seeing things—hallucinating. I explain her sensitivity to Gabapentin, and we agree to skip the next dose.

Then the nurse shifts gears. "Did she tell you about the bear?"

Convinced this is still part of Mom's delusional state, I roll my eyes. "Yes," I say, half amused, half exasperated. "She said she got it from the woman across the hall."

"That's actually true," the nurse replies. "I've been in nursing for thirty-five years, and I've never seen anything like it. Last night, your mom was really upset—crying out, inconsolable. The patient across the hall had a visitor who felt for her. She left, went to Target, and came back with that bear to comfort her."

We both paused, eyes misting over, caught in the quiet grace of that gesture.

Mom looked up and said, "See? I told you. I wasn't crazy."

Don't shy away from eye contact or small gestures of kindness—especially in a hospital. No one wants to be there. Sleep is elusive, and patients are constantly being poked, prodded, and repositioned as medical teams work to diagnose and treat their conditions. Look up. Look around. Offer a smile, hold a door, share a moment of grace. In a place filled with uncertainty and discomfort, a simple act of kindness can ripple farther than you'll ever know.

Hours blur together as we zone out, staring at the TV. First, we watch a documentary on safari animals, then a rerun of *The Price is Right*. Mom rambles about the contestant's too-short dress, then wonders aloud how old the host must be by now.

Without warning, she shifts into a story; one unfolding entirely in her mind. She starts talking about old friends she and Dad used to spend time with, recalling a shopping trip the four of them took to Home Depot. I have no idea where the memory is going or whether it's even real.

I don't interrupt. Instead, I listen. Every so often, I ask a gentle question, hoping to coax out more details, to follow the thread of whatever scene she's replaying. It's part memory, part imagination—and all hers.

It might feel instinctively kind to gently correct a loved one during a hallucination to tell them what they're seeing or experiencing isn't real. But that approach often does more harm than good. Especially in cases linked to dementia, hallucinations are vivid, present experiences unfolding in the person's mind. They can't distinguish between what's real and what's imagined. To them, it is real. And challenging that perception can lead to confusion, distress, or even fear. Compassionate validation, meeting them where they are, is often the more supportive path.

After several minutes, the hallucination dissipates, and she is back in the hospital room. She shifts to a fear-driven panic.

"Kath. I'm dizzy. I feel like I'm falling," she says.

I quietly move to the other side of the bed. Her eyes are closed, her brow tense with worry. I reach for her hand and hold it gently, anchoring her in the moment, hoping my presence will steady what her body and mind cannot.

"You're okay. You're not going to fall. You're lying in your bed."

"No, I'm not," she says, panic rising. "I'm going to fall."

I move closer, soften my voice. "Mom, you're safe. I promise. You trust me, right?"

"Yes," she whispers.

"I've never lied to you, have I?"

"No."

"I know it feels real, but you're in bed. You're not standing."

Her brow tightens. Tears stream down her cheeks. "I believe you," she says, breathless, "but that's not what's happening. I'm going to fall."

I try a new approach. "Do you see the chair behind you?"

"Yes."

"Bend your knees and sit back."

"I can't," she says, gripping my hand tighter. "I'm going to fall."

I return to the original strategy. "You're in bed. You're safe. You trust me, don't you?"

"Yes. I just don't understand why I feel like this."

She grows quiet. I dim the lights and mute the TV. Minutes pass. I watch the clock. Her tears continue, silent and steady.

Finally, her eyes open. "Kath, I believe you. I understand what you're saying. I really do. I ask God to help me—to help me see what's real—and I still see myself standing. I'm afraid of falling. Why would He do that?"

I cry. *I can't do this.* "Mom, I don't know," I say. "I wish I had a better answer. You're safe."

That's all I can offer. It's as if she's levitating. *Is she dying? Is this what it feels like?* I'm scared. Sad. Unnerved. I kiss her on the forehead and say, "I love you. I'll see you tomorrow." And I leave.

The next morning, I brace myself for more confusion, more fear. But when I walk into her room, she's sitting upright, finishing breakfast, smiling. Lucid. Chatting like nothing happened.

Just like that, she's back. She's normal again.

PureWick Explained: A Non-Invasive Option

I spend most of the day at Mom's bedside, keeping her company and watching for any signs of change. At one point, I notice a canister mounted to the wall behind her headboard. It's filled with fluid the color of weak tea. *That can't be good.*

I know what it is—it's the receptacle that collects urine from her external catheter, a PureWick. Picture a banana-sized, cotton-filled device with a hose attached, positioned between the legs. As the patient urinates, the cotton absorbs the fluid, and the hose pulls it away into the wall-mounted container.

But why is the fluid so dark? It should be pale yellow or clear. My mind jumps to kidney failure. I know that when the kidneys aren't properly flushing toxins, urine can turn darker. Concerned, I ask the next tech who enters the room. She's unsure and calls in the nurse.

The nurse reassures me: "Her kidneys are fine. What you're seeing is a mix of urine and stool from a recent bowel movement. We'll get her cleaned up."

It's a relief, but also a reminder of how complex and delicate elder care can be.

A urinary wicking device like a PureWick—or similar—is a practical solution designed to collect urine using absorption or gentle suction. It helps keep fluid from pooling, which can irritate the skin and lead to rashes or bedsores. Unlike indwelling (internal) catheters, these wicking devices are less invasive and offer greater comfort. They also provide more freedom of movement and independence compared to traditional options like bedpans.

Positioned externally, over or near the vulva, wicking devices absorb urine as it's released and channel it away, helping to prevent leaks and protect the skin from irritation. They're a practical solution for non-ambulatory patients, balancing dignity with function.

Rehab Services in Long-Term Care: What to Expect When Living There Permanently

When Mom is discharged and ready to return to her room at the long-term care facility, I have two concerns. One, can she go back to her room at the nursing home and if she does, will Medicare cover it because she's being discharged to rehab? And two, how do I get the hospital to coordinate her return transport via ambulance, and again, will Medicare cover it?

When a Medicare patient is discharged from the hospital and requires medically necessary rehabilitation, Medicare typically covers the cost of services like physical therapy (PT), occupational therapy (OT), and speech therapy. It also covers up to twenty-one days of housing in a rehab facility—fully, if the criteria are met.

Here's the dilemma: Mom lives in a long-term care facility where she has a permanent, privately paid room. We pay a significant monthly fee for her to receive 24/7 care. Within the same facility, there's a separate wing designated for skilled nursing rehab—where short-term patients recovering from surgeries like knee replacements receive care covered by Medicare.

Medicare's coverage structure is clear: 100 percent of costs are covered for the first twenty-one days in a skilled nursing rehab setting. From day twenty-two through day one hundred, Medicare pays a portion, and supplemental insurance may cover the rest.

So here's the question: Does she need to temporarily relocate to the skilled nursing rehab wing for Medicare to kick in? Or can she return to her permanent room and still qualify for coverage? And if she *can* return to her regular room, will the facility's billing office know to submit the claim to Medicare correctly?

We don't want to miss out on twenty-one days of covered care because of a clerical oversight. And we certainly don't want Medicare to flag her permanent residency as a reason to deny the claim. She's being discharged from the hospital into skilled nursing care—it just happens to be at the same facility where she already lives.

As any good project manager would, I'm thinking through the "what ifs." Because in elder care, the fine print matters—and so does the follow-through.

> **Inpatient Rehab Medicare Coverage**
> For those requiring inpatient rehabilitation after a hospital
> stay, a skilled nursing facility (SNF) is often the go-to option.
> In 2026, Medicare covers up to 100 days of rehab in an SNF
> per benefit period, subject to certain conditions:

- Days 1-20: You won't pay anything for your SNF stay, provided you've met the Part A deductible.

- Days 21-100: You'll be responsible for a daily coinsurance payment, determined by Medicare.

- Day 101 and beyond: You'll be responsible for covering the entire cost of your stay.

After several rounds of back-and-forth with the long-term care facility and the hospital social worker, our questions are finally answered. Mom can return to her permanent room, and Medicare will cover the first twenty-one days following her hospital discharge. No need for a temporary move to the skilled nursing wing.

From there, we keep a close eye on the invoices over the next few months, double-checking that we aren't mistakenly billed as private pay for the portion Medicare is supposed to cover.

Getting Home from the Hospital: The Private Ambulance Option

With hospital discharge arrangements in place, my attention shifts to the next logistical hurdle: transporting Mom from the hospital back to the nursing home. Her initial transfer was an emergency—911 was called due to low oxygen levels, labored breathing, and hallucinations. Now, with her UTI under control and discharge plans in motion, the question is: how do we get her back safely?

Mom is fully lift-dependent. She can't walk. She can barely sit upright without tipping over. The hospital social worker's suggestion? "You'll drive her back."

Absolutely not!

I'm a devoted daughter, but I'm not equipped to lift, stabilize, or transport someone in Mom's condition.

"We'll help you load her here," the social worker offers, "and the nursing home staff can assist when you arrive."

Still no.

Mom's anxiety, chronic pain, and panic, especially in a car, make that plan a recipe for disaster.

"We need to arrange a private ambulance transfer," I insist.

What follows is a tense back-and-forth. The social worker tries to reassure me that most families handle this themselves. I do my best to stay calm, but I'm firm. This isn't a matter of convenience; it's about safety.

Knowing I'm pushing my luck, I ask a critical question, "How do we ensure Medicare covers the cost of a private ambulance? Is there a specific billing code that needs to be included to show that private transport is medically necessary?"

"I don't know," she snips. "You'll have to contact Medicare about that."

Of course I will. Why would she try to help me figure this out? Another task on my to do list: play Medicare phone-tree tag until I find the last standing, *"not-it"* person who can answer my question. Will Medicare cover private ambulance transport from the hospital back to the nursing home? The answer I get is yes. In this case, Medicare *should* cover the service. Success. Now we just need to watch the next few months' medical claims to make sure everything gets paid.

Medicare Part B covers ambulance services in emergencies, and in certain cases, for non-emergency situations as well. If the transport is scheduled and the patient's health isn't in immediate jeopardy, it's not classified as an emergency. However, Medicare may cover non-emergency ambulance trips that are unscheduled or medically necessary, especially if the patient resides in a skilled nursing facility (SNF). In these cases, a doctor's written order is typically required within forty-eight hours of the transport to qualify for coverage.

With the private ambulance arranged, Medicare coverage confirmed, and an assurance that Mom can return to her permanent room at the nursing home (also covered under her plan) she is officially discharged. The latest crisis is averted, and I am free to fly back home tomorrow.

I wish I could have spent the Easter holiday with my immediate family, but as with most memories, I don't realize its impact until much later. That Easter weekend was one of my most memorable. I'm grateful for the kind visitor across the hall who bought a teddy bear after hearing Mom cry out in pain. I'm blessed to have visited my last surviving aunt and her children. I'm thankful I could join a high school friend and her family for Easter dinner. And afterward, I joined one of Mom's neighbor's for coffee. My greatest gift? Mom and I shared her final Easter together.

CHAPTER 17

Beyond Bingo— Creative Alternatives for Engaging Elders

Topics

— Here Comes the Bride …and Groom and the Parade of Wheelchairs

— Planning a Wedding Mom Can Attend

— A Reception Designed with Elders in Mind

— Ask, Listen, Learn: Unlocking Wisdom Sitting Beside You

— Christmas Lights and Cookie Tins: A Trip of a Lifetime

My Mom's generation might seem meek now, shuffling around nursing home hallways or crocheting baby hats, but these elders came of age in a time of upheaval. The sexual revolution was in full swing, and the birth control pill had just hit the market. They weren't just watching history unfold; they were making it.

Many ran households on shoestring budgets, raising children, sewing clothes, and stretching every dollar. Spa days and gym memberships weren't part of the equation. Some clocked in at factories, offices, or department stores. Others took on roles that demanded grit. One of Mom's housemates, Dee, swears like a sailor—and, from her perspective, she earned the right. She spent her career dispatching for the St. Louis Police Department. "I talked like the guys did," she says, grinning. "I fit in. They respected me. I was one of them." These women were tough, resourceful, and often rebellious long before anyone labeled them frail or fading.

Being mindful of long-term care residents' early lives, we can reimagine activities and experiences they may still enjoy. They don't want to sit idly by waiting to die, though many will say it feels that way. Despite physical limitations, they still find joy in gardening, crafting, movement, and mental stimulation. They want to feel engaged, not sidelined. Finding creative, meaningful ways to immerse elders in the world around them—not as spectators but as participants—honors their stories and keeps their skills and spirit alive.

Here Comes the Bride and Groom and the Parade of Wheelchairs

Despite history unfolding around her—bra burnings, Woodstock and protests—Mom chose to play it safe. Blocking it all out, she stayed inside her safe, suburban housewife bubble. Part of that was fear, but part of it was a craving for stability she'd never known as a child. Regardless of the reason, her orbit rarely stretched beyond a five-mile radius, with Aldi and Discount Liquor marking the outer limits of her perimeter.

Even in middle age, travel was the exception, not the norm. A visit to Michigan to see her best friend, or a trip to Texas to spend time with her grandkids, happened only occasionally. Flying was out of the question. Her claustrophobia was too intense. And highway driving sparked panic attacks. But for special occasions, like a grandson's birthday or Heritage Day at the elementary school when grandparents were celebrated, she'd push past the fear and make the journey from St. Louis. Even with Dad behind the wheel, she white-knuckled it the whole way.

Now, even those rare trips are out of reach because her health won't allow it. Travel is simply too strenuous, and the thought of missing her oldest grandson's wedding breaks her heart—and mine.

So, I craft a solution: we will bring the nuptials to Mom.

Planning a Wedding Mom Can Attend

A few months before Adam and Meagan's wedding, I reach out to two videographers—one in Texas, one in Missouri. The role of the Texas specialist (not the one hired to film the bride and groom's big moments) will live stream the ceremony. As Meagan walks down the aisle and vows are exchanged, Mom and her nursing home family in Missouri will be able to experience the wedding in real-time, watching it all unfold, moment by moment.

In Missouri, we hire a second videographer to manage the on-site technical setup. His role is to coordinate with the Texas team, ensuring the stream launches smoothly and without a hitch. A few weeks before the wedding, I make a quick trip to St. Louis to run a full tech rehearsal—testing internet speed, confirming Wi-Fi access, and checking for any firewall issues that might disrupt the live stream. Working out the tech kinks ahead of time means one less thing to worry about on the big day, and one more way to bring Mom into the heart of it all.

As part of my Missouri tech-testing trip, I also pack a large suitcase filled with wedding decorations and centerpiece supplies. We're bringing the wedding to the nursing home, and part of the joy is including the residents in the planning process.

The elders gather around the long kitchen table, eager to contribute. I pass out Polaroid candids of the bride and groom, and each resident clips the photos to a string using miniature clothespins. The task is more than just a sweet way to introduce them to the couple; it's also a valuable occupational therapy exercise, as they pinch the clips open and carefully fasten each image.

After the photo activity, we move on to table decorations. We fill plastic vases with clear beads and arrange white artificial hydrangeas. Wilma, one of the residents and the unofficial "house mom," takes charge. I create a multi-page instruction guide just for her, detailing how to set each table with a disposable tablecloth and gold place settings.

Giving Wilma a role gives her purpose. She becomes the director of transformation, leading staff and residents in turning the nursing home into a wedding reception filled with pride, beauty, and belonging.

For elders, having a purpose isn't just meaningful; it's vital. Purpose fuels dignity, connection, and vitality, especially in long-term care settings where routines can feel repetitive and isolating. When elders are invited to contribute, create, or lead, they're reminded that they still matter, not just as recipients of care, but as participants in life.

Why Engagement Matters for Elders

- **Cognitive engagement**: Purposeful tasks stimulate memory, attention, and problem-solving, helping slow cognitive decline.

- **Emotional well-being**: Feeling useful reduces depression, anxiety, and the sense of being a burden.

- **Physical health**: Activities with meaning—gardening, decorating, mentoring—encourage movement and dexterity.

- **Social connection**: Purpose often involves others, fostering relationships and reducing loneliness.

- **Identity preservation**: Roles like house mom, storyteller, or project lead help elders retain a sense of self beyond their diagnosis or limitations.

A Reception Designed with Elders in Mind

In addition to decorating the space, we arrange a senior-friendly meal from a local Italian restaurant and order a layered white wedding cake from Wal-Mart. A local musician plays familiar favorites, filling the room with joy and nostalgia.

We even replicate the wedding invitation, tailoring it for the nursing home. Instead of listing ceremony times, cocktail hour, and reception details, these invitations feature extra-large font for easier reading and warmly invite residents to witness a special event: Marlene's grandson marrying his bride, streamed live from Texas. Their communal living room, which we've transformed into a reception hall, becomes the heart of the celebration.

On the wedding day, all of Mom's housemates are pampered with fresh manicures, each one choosing her favorite shade of nail polish. We bring in a beautician who specializes in elder hair textures and techniques, ensuring every resident feels radiant.

The staff dresses Mom in her wedding outfit, a black lace sweater and matching pants bought just for this occasion. They add the finishing touch, a hand-delivered, beautiful wrist corsage to complete the outfit. Wilma decorates Mom's wheelchair with white balloons and streamers, transforming it into a seat of honor. Mom takes her place in the front row of the living room, ready to watch the ceremony unfold live.

Absorbed in the moment from my front-row pew, watching Adam and Meagan exchange vows, my phone buzzes. It's a text from one of the nursing home care partners—a photo of Mom. She looks stunning. Her makeup is flawless, her hair softly styled, her bubble-bath pink nails gleaming beneath the corsage. Her eyes are brimming with tears, and so are mine.

We did it. We brought the wedding to her. She's not an afterthought. She's not missing out. She's here—celebrating with us, surrounded by her nursing home family in Missouri.

Think beyond bingo and crafts. What real-world, hands-on experiences can you bring into long-term care to spark purpose and connection? Invite residents to pack toiletry kits for a local shelter, knowing their efforts will land in someone's hands that very night. Have them knit baby hats or booties for a crisis pregnancy center.

Adapt familiar games—corn hole, air hockey, ring toss—into movement-friendly versions that invite laughter, engagement and a touch of friendly competition.

You're not just planning activities. You're creating moments of meaning.

Find fresh, meaningful ways to engage aging loved ones. They don't want to sit on the sidelines watching time pass them by. They want to participate, contribute, and feel connected to what's happening. Invite them into the planning of holiday gatherings or charitable projects. Tap into their ideas, their lived experience, and their practical wisdom.

This is a generation of resourceful problem solvers. They've navigated life's complexities and still have so much to offer. Give them roles that matter. Let them lead, advise, create. Leveraging their talents and learning from them restores their sense of purpose, reminding them they are still valued and needed.

Ask, Listen, Learn: Unlocking Wisdom Sitting Beside You

A room full of history lessons is sitting right in front of me. I just need to engage. Who needs the 'grocery store' encyclopedias that Mom worked so hard to earn by collecting Blue Chip Stamps, when I'm sitting in a room full of living history born between 1930 and 1940?

Skip the dusty encyclopedias, the YouTube documentaries, and the late-night Googling of 'Agent Orange.' Just pull up a chair and talk to the residents at Mom's nursing home. Everyone, no matter their age, lights up when asked to share their own stories.

A single question can shift the conversation from aches and ailments to memories and meaning. These elders are living archives, rich with firsthand accounts of history, resilience, and everyday brilliance. All it takes is curiosity—and a little time.

> **Looking for conversation starters? Consider starting with these:**
>
> - Ask about their childhood home—what it looked like, who lived there, and what made it special.
>
> - If they grew up on a farm, explore the kinds of tools and equipment they used, and how daily chores shaped their routines.
>
> - Talk about school days. Did they wear uniforms? How big was their class? What subjects were taught in high school?

- Invite reflections on wartime memories—experiences with the draft, the return of veterans, or the spirit of patriotism in their community.

- Explore major news events from their youth, and how things like cost of living or world affairs shaped their perspective.

- Ask about favorite bands, radio shows, or early television programs that brought joy or sparked imagination.

As conversations with Mom's housemates unfold, remarkable stories surface. One resident has been married four times, another once led nursing operations at a level-one trauma hospital, and another was a World War II concentration camp survivor.

These exchanges aren't just interviews; they're invitations. A simple question can unlock a memory, offering residents a chance to revisit meaningful chapters of their lives. In sharing, they feel seen, valued, and heard, and I walk away honored and enriched. Our time sharing is a mutual gift: a lesson in resilience and humanity for one, and a moment of dignity and connection for the other.

Sensitivity matters. If a topic stirs discomfort or agitation, gently pivot to something lighter—a favorite meal, a sports team, or a recent event. For those living with dementia or Alzheimer's, recalling distant memories may be easier than short-term ones, especially in early and middle stages. But, if a distant memory is inaccessible, trying to remember it can bring frustration or confusion. In these moments, presence and patience speak louder than any question.

Christmas Lights and Cookie Tins: A Trip of a Lifetime

Another way to engage nursing home housemates is to change things up and plan an outing. Some facilities offer off-property field trips, while others may not. But this doesn't mean meaningful excursions are off the table.

One year, when we took Mom to see Christmas lights, I swore I'd never do it again. Then I discovered a better option. Instead of maneuvering

Mom into my nephew's sedan, I rented a wheelchair accessible van, which was a game-changer.

These vehicles—often called wheelchair vans, mobility vans, or conversion vans—are designed specifically for individuals with physical impairments. Features like ramps, lowered floors, wide doors, and secure tie-down systems make entering and exiting safe and dignified. Adjustable seating adds comfort, turning what could otherwise feel like logistical Jenga into what it should be: a smooth, enjoyable outing, sharing time together.

After learning my lesson from the earlier "surprise" visit, when Mom 'forgot' how to bend her body and resisted being helped into a car, I decide to give her a heads-up this time. No last-minute plans, no scrambling. Instead, I tell her in advance: "We're planning a field trip. First stop: Dollar Tree for Christmas shopping. Then, we'll drive through the park to see the lights and grab pizza on the way back. How does that sound?"

"Great," she says. And our plan is in motion.

The Dollar Tree shopping spree is a treasured memory. We spent nearly two hours roaming the aisles. Mom "suddenly" remembered she needed a room deodorizer, fingernail polish, and a new broom. She hand-picked Christmas cards for each family member and chose festive towels and cookie tins for her nursing home friends.

We sang Christmas carols at full volume as we drove to the city park, where the local Lions Club had sponsored a dazzling light display. On the way back, we picked up her favorite pizza and a six-pack of beer.

I wouldn't trade that Christmas for anything. It was filled with love, laughter, and peace. And I'm especially grateful for it now, knowing it turned out to be our last Christmas together.

CHAPTER 18

Cognitive Decline— Is it Time for Memory Care?

Topics

— Cognitive Decline: What to Look For

— Memory Boosters: Aids for Aging Minds

— Understanding Dementia: A Closer Look at the Different Types

— Strategies for Supporting Someone Living with Mental Decline

— Memory Care: What Makes It Different

Back in the 1950s, high schoolers weren't glued to screens and wearing out their thumbs texting. Instead, they mastered their own cryptic language: shorthand. With its dots, dashes, and squiggles, shorthand was a staple of the secretarial curriculum, taught alongside typing class and bookkeeping. Some elders still carry these skills today, able to read and write in this forgotten language.

At first, finding pages of mom's old steno pad filled with shorthand might bring up feelings of a charming throwback. But realizing she's using it to record every detail of a visit—what was said, what she felt, what she wants to remember—that raises less nostalgia and more concern. Her notes aren't just reflections; they're anchors. And that quiet urgency in her scribbles may be telling a poignant story: it might be time to consider memory care.

The terms *dementia* and *Alzheimer's* have been around for over a century, and confusion between them has lasted just as long. But understanding the difference matters. In simple terms, dementia is the broader category, a general decline in cognitive function, while Alzheimer's is its most common form, accounting for 60-80 percent of cases. [Source: *Dementia vs. Alzheimer's: How to Tell the Difference*, aarp.org]

As dementia progresses, an elder may struggle with activities of daily living, experience shifts in mood or behavior and even face delusions or hallucinations. Noticing early changes, understanding when safety may be at risk, and intervening when needed are central to supporting the aging journey.

Cognitive Decline: What to Look For

Mom lives with a long list of physical ailments, chronic pain, and mental health challenges. She also has her share of hallucinations and delusional moments. Her hallucinations and delusions come and go, and they're often intensified by something as common as a urinary tract infection, which research shows affects older women more frequently than men.

We've witnessed Mom's 'off' behavior multiple times from gallon ice cream lids filled with milk for imaginary cats and dogs she swears are roaming the kitchen, to moments in her hospital bed where she seems to levitate as she describes looking down on long ago memories with Dad and friends, who passed away years ago. These episodes are heartbreaking reminders that her mind doesn't always hold steady. Dementia slips in, and reality slips away.

Mom doesn't have Alzheimer's, but my grandmother wasn't as fortunate. Within a year, she slid from managing independently in a senior living facility to being placed in what was then called a mental institution, long before the term *memory care* was coined.

The transition was brutal. For the safety of staff and other patients, my grandmother was heavily medicated. Doses so strong they left her in a near-catatonic state. I still remember her slumped in a wheelchair, eyes vacant, surrounded by the sterile hum of a locked ward. It wasn't care. It was containment.

It Started with a Trip to the Convenience Store

The first signs that my grandmother's mind was slipping came after we'd moved to Texas. I was newly married, juggling full-time work and raising two toddlers. Between daycare costs, college savings, and trying to be super parents, our lives were full. Trips back to St. Louis were rare.

Then, on a cold Wednesday in January, my dad called. His voice was solemn. "Gardy isn't doing well," he said.

Gardy was our family nickname—one that started when my sister couldn't quite pronounce "grandma"—and it stuck. Sweet, simple, and now suddenly heavy.

"What do you mean she's not doing well?" I asked.

"I was over at her apartment about a week ago, and she looked me straight in the eye, serious as she could be, and said, 'Joe, I was sitting here watching TV, and clear as day, Matthew walked right through that wall. It was the darndest thing I've ever seen.'"

"That's not all of it," he continued. "I sort of ignored it, thinking she's just talking crazy. But then I got a call at two in the morning from the police. They were at the convenience store with her. She said she was buying cigarettes for her husband. She said she got confused and didn't know how to get home."

Getting home was just one of her problems. Her husband had been dead for twenty-five years. My dad went on to explain how he got her back home and took her car keys. That moment marked the beginning of a steep mental decline. Within a year, Gardy was gone.

But in those last months, my Mom fought tirelessly to find her a safe place to stay, one facility after another. Each time, shortly after getting her settled, Gardy would be evicted for lashing out at staff, taking things that weren't hers, or getting into physical altercations with other residents.

She wasn't herself. She was mad, scared, and confused. Her mind was slipping, and we were watching it happen in real time.

My last memory of her is etched in stillness: heavily sedated, resting in a nursing home bed barely six inches off the ground. It was a quiet end for a woman who had once radiated innocence. She loved having her nails done, her hair curled and wearing the most stylish outfits her modest budget could afford. She was always put together—elegant, expressive, and full of wonder.

She saw the world through the eyes of a child. Clouds were puffy cotton balls. Christmas morning lit her up more than any three-year-old. And she loved playing board games at the kids' table. That spark, so uniquely hers, lingered even as her body and mind faded.

Memory Boosters: Aids for Aging Minds

What You Can Do to Support Brain Health

Even if your loved one isn't showing signs of decline, these strategies can help protect cognitive function and may slow progression if symptoms are emerging:

- **Keep the mind active**: Encourage puzzles, reading, storytelling, or learning something new.

- **Stay physically engaged**: Daily walks, stretching, or light exercise can boost blood flow to the brain.

- **Eat for brain health**: A Mediterranean-style diet rich in vegetables, fish, and healthy fats supports cognitive resilience.

- **Prioritize sleep**: Poor sleep can mimic or worsen memory issues.

- **Manage chronic conditions**: High blood pressure, diabetes, and heart disease are linked to cognitive decline.

- **Foster emotional well-being**: Stress, isolation, and depression can accelerate memory loss.

- **Stay socially connected**: Regular interaction helps preserve memory and mood.

The earliest signs of forgetfulness can be subtle or jarring. One day, an aging parent seems perfectly fine, like my grandmother. The next, they're repeating questions, misplacing familiar items, or acting in ways that feel strangely out of character. But when these moments begin to multiply, shift in tone, or come with emotional changes like anxiety, withdrawal, or frustration, it may be time to look closer. Early signs of cognitive decline can be easily overlooked, and they don't always point to Alzheimer's or dementia. Sometimes, they're reversible. Sometimes, they're not. Either way, noticing them early can help with a diagnosis and treatment plan, if available.

Early Warning Signs to Watch For:

- *Repeating questions or stories within short timeframes*

- *Difficulty following conversations or instructions*

- *Confusion about time, place, or familiar routines*

- *Mood swings, irritability, or withdrawal from social activities*

- *Trouble managing finances, medications, or appointments*

- *Unusual behaviors like writing detailed notes to remember conversations*

Understanding Dementia: A Closer Look at the Different Types

Dementia may present differently depending on the person, and even within the broad category of dementia, there are various forms—vascular dementia, Alzheimer's disease, mixed dementia, and others. But regardless of the type, it brings heartache for both the person experiencing it and the loved ones trying to make sense of the changes.

Vascular Dementia - Caused by damage to blood vessels in the brain, leading to cognitive decline.

Frontotemporal Dementia - Affects the frontal and temporal lobes of the brain, causing changes in personality, behavior, and language.

Alzheimer's Disease - The most common type of dementia, characterized by progressive memory loss, confusion, and changes in behavior.

Mixed Dementia - A combination of two or more types of dementia, such as Alzheimer's and vascular dementia.

It's important to note that symptoms and progression of dementia can vary depending on the specific type. A healthcare professional can help diagnose and determine the best course of treatment. Consult a physician about available medications. While some drugs can help manage symptoms and slow the progression, they don't stop, reverse, or provide a cure for the underlying disease. The effectiveness of medications used to temporarily improve cognitive symptoms can vary, with improvements often lasting six to twelve months.

Medications for dementia fall into two major categories:

- **Cholinesterase inhibitors**: These drugs boost levels of acetylcholine, a chemical messenger important for memory and judgment, by preventing its breakdown in the brain. Examples include donepezil (Aricept), rivastigmine (Exelon), and galantamine. They are often used for mild-to-moderate Alzheimer's disease and may also benefit those with Lewy body or Parkinson's disease dementia.

- **Memantine (Namenda)**: This drug regulates the activity of glutamate, another brain chemical involved in learning and memory. It is prescribed for moderate-to-severe Alzheimer's and is sometimes used in combination with a cholinesterase inhibitor.

A friend recently shared a story about her mother, who had just been diagnosed with vascular dementia. It brought tears to my eyes.

When Celebrating Your Birthday Makes You Cry

You feel the sadness settle in when the lemon chiffon cake—your birthday tradition for forty years is suddenly just... gone. Mom doesn't remember the recipe. She doesn't even remember that lemon chiffon was your favorite.

You've reminded her gently, over and over during the past twenty minutes: You're here to celebrate your birthday.

"Oh, I'm sorry, dear," she says. "Of course it's your birthday. I forgot. I need to get you a gift."

There's a pause. Silence stretches across the room. Her eyes glaze over. You brace yourself.

"Hi, dear. Who are you?"

It hits like a punch to the gut. You steady your voice and remind her *again* that you're her daughter. And you're here to celebrate your birthday with her.

Another friend, reflecting on the challenges of caring for her aging mother, shared a story that still haunts me. Her mom hadn't been mentally sharp for some time, but she had just enough clarity and determination to craft a plan to hide her decline.

It wasn't until months after settling her mother into a memory care facility that my friend uncovered the truth. While cleaning out the house to prepare it for sale, she opened a bedroom dresser drawer and found a stack of steno pads—white, pink, and blue. They were relics from her mother's secretarial days in the '70s.

She began flipping through them, ready to toss them aside until something made her pause. *These weren't old work notes. They were transcripts.* Her mother had recorded detailed accounts of their visits: who got married, who passed away, what degree her grandson was pursuing, what month it was, what holiday was coming next.

Some pages were written in shorthand, filled with squiggles and dots. Others were composed in perfect penmanship, full sentences laid out with care.

My friend cried. The realization hit hard: her mother had been scared, confused, and desperate to hold on. Too timid to admit she was slipping, she'd quietly documented every conversation, reconstructing their time together, line by line, just to remember.

"She was terrified of being found out," my friend said. "Writing it all down was her way of coping. It must have taken her hours to recreate our dialogue."

Strategies for Supporting Someone Living with Mental Decline

Helping an aging parent navigate cognitive changes requires both empathy and adaptability. What feels frustrating to the care team can be equally distressing for the person experiencing memory loss. Visual cues and environmental support can ease confusion, reduce anxiety, and foster a sense of independence.

- **Large Calendar** - Place a large, easy-to-read calendar in a prominent location like the refrigerator or near the front door. Include doctor's appointments, physical therapy sessions, birthdays, and holidays. Seeing the day, date, and upcoming events at a glance can help orient someone who struggles to track time.

- **Whiteboard or Dry-Erase Board** - Use a whiteboard to list essential phone numbers—neighbors, caregivers, family members. And update it regularly. This not only provides quick access for the elder but also helps others who may be assisting. It's a visual cue that reinforces connection and safety.

- **Labels and Signs** - Label drawers, cabinets, and rooms with large-print signs (e.g., "Toothbrush," "Snacks," "Bathroom") to reduce confusion and support independence. Use photos alongside words for added clarity. This is especially helpful for elders with more advanced decline.

- **Photo Memory Wall** - Create a wall of labeled family photos with names and relationships (e.g., "Susan—

Daughter," "Ben—Grandson"). This can spark recognition and comfort. Include seasonal or holiday-themed photos to help orient them to the time of year.

- **Digital Clocks with Day and Date** - Invest in a digital clock that displays the time, day of the week, and full date. Some models also include reminders like "It's morning" or "Time for medication."

- **Medication Chart or Pill Organizer** - Use a visual medication chart with times and dosages, paired with a color-coded pill organizer. This helps reduce missed or repeated doses and supports routine.

- **Voice-Activated Assistants**—Devices like Alexa or Google Assistant can simplify daily tasks. Saying, "Alexa, add margarine to the shopping list," is a quick, hands-free way to keep track of groceries. These tools can also set reminders, play music, or answer simple questions, offering both utility and companionship.

- **Digital Picture Frame**—An alternative to a photo memory wall is a digital picture frame. A rotating slideshow of familiar faces, holidays, and favorite places can offer comfort and orientation. Whether placed on a countertop or bedside table, digital frames allow family members to remotely update photos and add captions with names of those in the photo, keeping the display fresh and meaningful.

- **Mobile Device Games**—If dexterity and vision allow, apps like Wordle, Crossword, or Sudoku can help keep the mind active. These games offer gentle cognitive stimulation and can be a fun part of a daily routine.

New technologies continue to emerge that help caregivers and aging parents navigate the challenges of declining memory. Yet as valuable as these tools can be, many older adults have never learned to use modern devices and may find them confusing or inaccessible. Flexibility and thoughtful accommodations are essential.

Tech Tips

Medication Reminders—*Use apps or smart pill dispensers that alert the elder when it's time to take medication.*

GPS Tracking—*For those prone to wandering, wearable devices or phone apps can provide peace of mind.*

Video Calling—*Regular virtual check-ins with family can reduce isolation and reinforce relationships.*

Apps for TV Remote Control—*Smartphone or tablet apps are available to control or 'fix' a broken TV remote control when mom presses a wrong button and can't change the channel.*

Smart Lighting—*Automated lights that adjust with time of day can help with sleep cycles and reduce confusion.*

Memory Care: What Makes It Different

Nurturing cognitive health calls for intentional, well-tailored strategies. Tools like voice assistants, digital calendars, and visual cues can reinforce routines and ease daily confusion. Yet as cognitive decline deepens, these supports may no longer suffice. When safety and independence can't be maintained, even with help, a transition to memory care may become essential.

Memory care is a specialized form of long-term care designed specifically for individuals with Alzheimer's disease, dementia, or other cognitive impairments. Providing a safe, structured setting that meets the evolving needs of those experiencing mental decline, memory care is typically housed in a dedicated wing or standalone unit within assisted living or skilled nursing communities.

Whether it happens gradually or all at once, watching a parent decline, mentally, physically, or both, is never easy. It's a delicate dance, trying to meet the needs of immediate family, manage work responsibilities, and show up fully for someone who once cared for you.

And as I move through this season of caregiving, I've become more attuned to the realities of aging, not just Mom's, but mine, as well. My knees creak a little more than they used to, I'm not as quick on my feet, and those reading glasses I used to reach for occasionally have become a permanent fixture on the bridge of my nose.

It's a stark reminder to realize that the care I offer today may be the same care I need tomorrow. But there's also clarity in this awareness—a deeper appreciation for the present, and a renewed commitment to show up with empathy, patience, and grace.

RESOURCES

Book: The 36-Hour Day: A Family Guide to Caring for People Who Have Alzheimer Disease, Other Dementias, and Memory Loss (A Johns Hopkins Press Health Book) April 18, 2017

By Nancy L. Mace (Author), Peter V. Rabins (Author)

CHAPTER 19

This is Hard—Is She Dying? Dealing with Decline

Topics

— Facing the Realities of Decline: What it Looks Like and How it Feels

— When Accidents Happen: The Truth About Incontinence and Bed Soiling

— The Meeting: On the Brink of Eviction

— Running on Empty: Caregiver Burnout is Numbing

The phrase "sh*t the bed" takes on a whole new meaning, and it's no longer a sarcastic or humorous quip when it becomes an aging parent's new reality.

Surprise! Soiling the bed is okay. Sometimes, it's the most practical option nursing staff can offer when mobility is gone. How degrading it must feel when hands no longer cooperate to wipe, scratch, brush, or feed. Dignity gets redefined. It's hard to imagine the emotional toll of losing control over basic functions when the body deteriorates ahead of the mind. Neurological decline and muscular dysmorphia affect the body when they settle in.

Facing the Realities of Decline: What it Looks Like and How it Feels

Man, this is hard. The kind of hard that has me jumping on a plane with no notice because Mom is being rushed to the ER. The kind that spikes my anxiety every time the caller ID on my phone flashes the name of the care facility. The kind that forces tense negotiations with my sister about what to do next. This stage is a *new* kind of hard. Mom is now a full-time resident in a long-term care facility. Her neuropathy continues its relentless assault on her nervous system. She can't walk, stand, or sit on the toilet. Her willpower still fuels her fight to feed herself—but even that's becoming a marathon. Eating a bowl of oatmeal takes two hours.

Her mind is sharp, engaged, and still very much *her*—until a UTI hits. Then, the hallucinations return. Cats, she swears, are traipsing across her room.

Each month, she loses a little more weight. Her body is fragile. She's been through so much. Her skin is almost translucent. Her face is more gray than pink. Is she dying? Yes. But when? Who knows?

The flurry of emotions I experience at each stage of this process is maddening. Some days I'm seething. Angry, exhausted, pushed to the edge. Other days, the sadness takes over. Watching her navigate such a stripped-down version of life is heartbreaking. This isn't the retirement she imagined. It's a slow erosion of independence, dignity, and joy. She feels defeated, reliant, and convinced she's a burden.

Mom's world has narrowed to two positions: in her wheelchair or lying in bed. The daily bingo game is her main event, but even that wears thin. There are only so many packs of Wrigley spearmint gum or tiny plush toys you can win before the novelty fades into monotony.

The woman has no core muscle strength. The neuropathy has infiltrated her body. We believe it has weakened her extremities and robbed them of most feeling. But there are times when we wonder how much of it is physical versus how much is mental. When she's asked to do something differently, Mom vehemently resists change. Anxiety floods in, convincing her she can't lift, grasp, or move, even when her body might still be capable. *Is she physically incapable or is her mind frozen, making her believe she can't do something?* Mom's low pain tolerance and her ability to differentiate discomfort from dislike are perpetually blurred lines.

We inherit traits from our parents—some we embrace, others we reject intensely. For me, the trait I'm most determined to break is Mom's lifelong habit of making excuses. It's one of the reasons why I bird-dog every detail of her care, why I push so hard for clarity, accountability, and action. Mom is the queen of "yes, but…" and I think that's part of why I'm so tough on myself. I try to name my own excuses when they show up. When I hear "I can't because…" in my head, I recognize it for what it is. Sometimes I push through and do the hard thing anyway. Other times, I eat. For some, it's alcohol or shopping. For me, it's food. That internal tennis match—between "I should" and "I don't want to"—plays out every time I procrastinate calling her.

Because calling her, visiting her, engaging with her–it's all hard. She's depressed. She's in pain. And she cries. A lot. No matter what we talk about, I try to lift the mood. But within moments, she's weeping, asking, "Why am I here? Why don't I just die? There's no point in living."

I respond with the usual comfort: "You're special. God has a reason for you being here." But the truth is, I wonder too. Her quality of life isn't what she wants or dreamed of. And, as she puts it, "I'm just existing. I'm not living."

She's not wrong. She's confined to a wheelchair or hospital bed, completely dependent on others to lift, position, and care for her. These aren't the golden years she imagined. I don't blame her for wanting out. Who would want to live like this?

But what's the alternative? I wish something could change for her, and for us. A tweak here, a med change there, a new therapeutic bed pillow. The list goes on. But none of it seems to matter. With no power to change it, she's enduring this prolonged, joyless chapter until her body finally gives out. It's heartbreaking. And it feels like we're all trapped in this vortex with her.

When Accidents Happen: The Truth About Incontinence and Bed Soiling

Because of Mom's progressive muscular atrophy and weakened core strength, she can no longer sit upright on the toilet. The alternative? A bedpan—awkward, uncomfortable, and far from ideal. It's well known that prolonged bedpan use increases the risk of bedsores, and with her paper-thin skin, this means inevitable tears, infections, and pain.

But as unpleasant as the bedpan is, I've discovered something worse: being told to soil the bed. That's exactly what the nursing facility instructed. *Just go in the bed.* As absurd as it sounds, it wasn't the first time. During her last hospital stay, the care team said the same thing: "We have to change her anyway. We'll just let her go in the bed."

I thought I'd seen it all. But pooping in your bed? A grown woman being told that's acceptable? My mom is mortified. Still, what choice does she have? Her dignity, pride, and modesty have been stripped away. If that's what the staff tells her to do, she complies.

This process feels barbaric. Inhumane. And I've developed a whole new weighted understanding for the phrase *"sh*t the bed."* It's no longer a cheeky way to describe a botched project or a mistake. Now, it evokes something literal, visceral, and deeply humiliating.

If an aging parent says they've been told to poop in bed, believe them. This practice occurs in hospitals and nursing homes. Ask questions. Find out how often patients are cleaned and changed afterward. Understand whether it's a standard protocol or simply the path of least resistance for an overworked shift. Dignity deserves advocacy.

The Meeting: On the Brink of Eviction

The long-term care facility calls an all-hands meeting—unusual, since it's typically Tina and I who initiate these. That alone raises red flags. I join from Texas via Zoom; Tina attends in person. Virtual meetings with the facility are always a technological circus. They use the free version of Zoom, so forty-five minutes in, we get booted off and spend another ten minutes trying to reconnect. But this time feels different. More organized. They've invited everyone: dietary staff, two care partners, the nurse on duty, the social worker, the activities director, the director of operations— plus Mom, Tina, and me.

Mom struggles with Zoom. She's getting used to it, but seeing herself on screen still unsettles her. She fixates on her drawn face, her limp hair and her reflection more than the conversation.

As usual, Kayla, director of nursing, starts with the obligatory question: "Do you still want the DNR in place?" And as usual, I bristle. *Really?* Every single time we meet, we ask this dying woman if she wants to be resuscitated. I get the legal requirement, but it feels cruel. She signed the paperwork. We discussed it when she was admitted. Let it be. Yes, people change their minds. But in Mom's case, death would be a relief. Merciful.

Once we move past the DNR ritual, the real reason for the meeting surfaces: Mom is misbehaving, and the staff is at a breaking point. They're out of ideas. No matter what they do, she's unhappy.

She's becoming a menace as she stirs up her housemates, rallying complaints and creating a mutiny against the staff. She presses her call button constantly, and when no one responds fast enough, she yells. When someone does show up, she either forgets why she called or lashes out at them for not doing their job "right."

Mom has favorites. If she senses a bad attitude or unfamiliarity, she turns hostile. She's like a shark sensing weakness. And unfortunately, she dislikes more staff members than she likes.

The latest issue is related to lifting her. She can no longer be lifted safely, even by two care partners. As a result, they've transitioned her to a Hoyer lift—a mechanical hoist. Picture a giant canvas sling, like the kind used to immobilize a broken arm. It's tucked under her in bed, then clipped to a ceiling-mounted ring. She's wrapped up like a taco and hoisted from horizontal to vertical, then lowered into her wheelchair.

Now imagine doing that several times a day with someone who screams, panics, and cries through every transfer. That's the staff's reality. And it's no wonder some have asked to be reassigned to another floor.

Our family meeting isn't just about logistics. It's about poor behavior, fear, control, and the slow erosion of dignity—for Mom and for those trying to care for her.

My sister and I sense the "We can't help her anymore" speech coming. Moving her somewhere else is not a choice. She's in a top-tier facility, and the staff is doing an exceptional job. She's formed connections, friendships with the women on her floor. Everyone, from the administrator to the housekeeping staff knows her. Starting over somewhere else would be unsettling and cruel. It's not an option.

Then comes the question: "Marlene, are you happy here?" It lands with a thud. Asking a woman who resents paying thousands of dollars a month to live in a place she loathes if she's happy feels tone-deaf. Tina snaps. Her frustration erupts. My shoulders tense, and nausea creeps in. Her outburst only escalates the tension.

The staff responds swiftly. One opens the wide glass door. Another releases the brake on Mom's wheelchair and gently rolls her out of the room, removing her from the emotional crossfire. I'm grateful. Mom may be difficult, stubborn, and sharp-tongued, but she's also vulnerable.

The tension in the room is thick. I, too, wish I could leave, but I can't. I try to restore order. As Mom's family, it's our responsibility to model civility. Together we must resolve the situation and find a viable solution.

While I find my sister's behavior disturbing and, at times, humiliating, I also recognize the emotional toll this journey has taken on all of us. We're exhausted. Mom is exhausted. We've poured countless hours and mental energy into navigating the complex, often unsatisfying terrain of elder care—with no clear end in sight.

> The constant demands of caring for aging parents can lead to stress, frustration, depression, and even moments of hopelessness. The emotional toll is real and deserves recognition. Caregivers may feel isolated, exhausted, or guilty for not being able to do more, even when you are already giving everything you have.
>
> Just as patients need medical care, caregivers need emotional support and compassion. Naming these struggles is not a sign of weakness—it is a step toward resilience. With the right resources, community, and acknowledgment, caregivers can find strength in their role and hope in knowing they are not alone.
>
> Resources such as counseling services, support groups and peer-networks are available.

> Caregiver Action Network (CAN): Provides resources, support, and access to counseling for caregivers.
>
> Family Caregiver Alliance: Offers educational materials, support groups, and counseling.
>
> NAMI (National Alliance on Mental Illness) Family-To-Family (education) and peer-led Family Support Groups for loved ones of those with mental illness.

Yes, Mom is dying. Her frailty is undeniable. Each visit reveals more: her cheeks hollower, her forehead more pronounced. It takes little imagination to glimpse the outline of the human skull beneath her skin. Her arms are now barely thicker than a tennis racket's shaft, and her toenails have grown thick, yellowed, and misshapen. But what options do we have? We must work with the staff, support her the best we can and look for a workable path forward.

If you are too emotional or enmeshed in a situation, recruit the support of a neutral party. This could be the nursing home social worker, a staff member at the facility, or a third-party family member. Leveraging an unbiased broker to calm an explosive situation can help mitigate conflict and refocus a meeting to move towards more constructive outcomes with actions and next steps.

Running on Empty: Caregiver Burnout is Numbing

I know I love my mom because I'm her daughter, because she raised me, because she showed up in all the ways a mother should. She did my laundry, helped me with spelling words, taught me to sew. She drove me and a car full of giggling tweens through McDonald's in her 1959 black Oldsmobile, which we proudly called the Batmobile. These memories are real, and they matter. But with each passing day, they are more distant, more blurred.

Now, what I see is someone who's resistant, anxious, and hard to be around. A woman who complains constantly, who is a stress-filled shadow of herself. She's living longer than she ever imagined, especially without Dad. She's sad. She's depressed. And with the weight of her mental health challenges and physical limitations, she's often miserable to be around. I know she doesn't want to be—but that doesn't change how hard it is.

Mom makes everything more complicated. Instead of looking forward to an outing, she finds reasons to avoid it. New aches and pains surface, triggering fresh waves of anxiety. Take, for example, one December when Tina and I took her out of the nursing home to see Christmas lights. What began as a joyful idea quickly unraveled. She forgot how to bend at the waist to help with the wheelchair transfer, and the evening ended with her choking on a piece of her favorite pizza.

Mom's anxiety turns even simple pleasures into high-stakes ordeals, and fun outings or field trips now fall into the "too hard" pile. I wish it were different. I wish she could embrace spontaneity and joy. But her fear takes over—and when it does, she takes me down with her.

Check your own expectations. This can be difficult, especially if you have an outing or special adventure planned. Even the most enthusiastic, go-with-the-flow elder can have an off day. Fatigue, pain, or anxiety may surface unexpectedly.

Be prepared: you might arrive at the facility only to find your parent isn't up for it. If the activity itself brings you joy, consider going anyway. But if the experience hinges on sharing it with your loved one, it's okay to postpone. Wait for a day when she's feeling stronger, more herself. Flexibility isn't just a kindness to her; it's a gift to you, too.

It's easy to be judgmental from the outside until you're living it yourself. I used to look at nursing homes and think, "How sad. These poor elders, abandoned by their families." I remember the Girl Scout field trips to the local facility, the awkward smiles, the sense of pity. But now, living this reality, I understand the deep, complicated pain that comes with caring for an aging parent.

No amount of festive door decorations or rounds of bingo, no ruby red lipstick or sparkly slippers can conjure the warmth and connection I once hoped for. The truth is that caregiving doesn't always feel like love. It feels like a duty. And whether we admit it or not, we all hope for something in return when we invest in relationships—maybe a listening ear, a spark of conversation, a moment of affection. Anything that reminds us that we're still seen. Whatever it is we are looking for, we desire a return on our investment.

For what feels like a lifetime, I've poured myself into caregiving—refilling my "Mom tank" again and again, searching for fresh energy and creative ways to meet each new challenge. But I'm drained. I don't want to do this anymore. All of it has aged me terribly. I don't want to call her. I don't want to visit her. I don't want to see her. I've developed a terrible case of the *I don't want to's*. I don't want to talk to any more caregivers or doctors. I don't even want to talk to my mother. Now, instead of calling her weekly, I can barely muster the energy to call her once every three weeks. I just want it over.

Is this normal? Yes. There are times during Mom's aging journey when I need to be in high-octane, project-management crisis mode, and then at other times, things are quiet. In the quiet times, there's no crisis of the moment, and I'm thankful. I feel less anxious. Relieved nothing needs to be solved today.

Living out of state adds a bittersweet layer. In the quiet stretches, I can mentally step back, almost pretend it's not happening. But that reprieve is fragile. At any moment, I can be pulled back to St. Louis—fast and forceful, like an overzealous lab on an afternoon walk. The unpredictability is exhausting.

This isn't a project with a clean arc. There's no final review, no tidy wrap-up, no Gantt chart to track progress. Managing Mom's care is like overseeing a project that never ends—and never improves. I imagine I'll cry when she passes. I'll feel the loss. But right now, it's hard to picture that moment clearly. I'm so depleted. I'm not just tired; I'm scraped thin. Struggling to summon compassion, even for the people I love. I'm beyond burnout; I'm hollow inside.

CHAPTER 20

What Is Hospice and Are We There Yet?

Topics

— A Trip to the ER: Something is Different This Time

— The Key Phrase That Opens the Door to Hospice

— Meeting the Hospice Intake Coordinator

— Clarifying Hospice: What It Offers—and What It Doesn't

Is Mom ready for hospice? I have no idea. Like every phase of this process, I'm improvising. Maybe we're already treating her like a hospice patient, just without the official label or the right Medicare billing code. And that raises a haunting question: is the definition of decline tied to how it's billed? It seems that way sometimes–most times.

From what I hear about hospice, what I read, I think I understand what they provide, but I get push back when trying to get it started with Mom. And push back comes from my sister and the doctor. I don't understand why. If Mom is dying and hospice is supposed to be this great resource to bring her comfort, why is the doctor who sees her every week at the nursing home refusing to order it? Even the staff who works with her daily suggest it, and still the doctor refuses. According to the nurse, "The doctor said you have to have less than six months to live for him to sign the paper, and your mom does not have an end-stage diagnosis."

I learn that each physician is different. And since hospice is a Medicare-covered service, that makes it government regulated. Plus, it's an expensive service, so regulations have tightened, and physicians are under great scrutiny. This is unfortunate because patients suffer. Mom can benefit from hospice services such as more frequent bathing (the nursing home bathes her twice a week, and hospice services augment this with an additional bath each week). Hospice care can also give her additional nursing support with bandage changes when she gets sores on her legs and repositioning her, whether shifting in her bed or navigating from her wheelchair to a recliner.

In the interim, we continue with our own comfort solutions from technology — her Alexa responding to Mom's voice command to "Play Kenny Rogers, *Through the Years*"; to a social companion who visits a few evenings each week just to talk, comb her hair, and help with watering her plants. She also refreshes the door wreath and room decorations for the upcoming holiday. All small attempts at making her final days, months, years bearable.

A Trip to the ER: Something is Different This Time

I receive an early-morning emergency call, something that I never quite get used to. It's the night nurse. She thinks Mom had a stroke. Her speech is slurred, and she's semi-coherent. The nurse explains that they've called 911, and the ambulance is on its way. Since there are Do Not Resuscitate (DNR) orders on file, the nurse needs to confirm if we want her transported or if we want her to remain at the nursing home. I said, "Yes. Send her to the hospital. Let's see what's going on."

Back to St. Louis I return. The routine is familiar, but never comfortable. Throw shirts, jeans, socks, underwear into a suitcase. Grab a set of workout clothes, just in case I find the time or motivation to use them, and I head to the airport. I'm not sure why, but I sense this isn't the usual situation where they discover a raging UTI, give her some antibiotics and fluids, and then send her back to the nursing home, business as usual. This time, I sense something different.

Tina picks me up at our usual spot, and we head to the hospital. The doctor has already ruled out a stroke. He is now testing for a UTI, and because she's complaining of severe stomach pain, he's also ordered an upper and lower GI to see what's going on. As we race down the highway, Tina gets a call. I overhear muffled phrases coming from the nurse on the other end.

"Oh, the doctor is there," Tina responds. "They are ready to take her back for the procedure?"

I blurt out, "No!" My eyes fill with tears. I plead. "I want to see her before they put her under anesthesia, please."

Tina hands me the phone. I pick up the conversation with the nurse. "Hi. This is Marlene's other daughter. I want to see her before she goes under," I beg. "Please wait until we get there. I just flew in. I don't live here."

The nurse agrees to move another patient's case up, delaying the procedure so I can get there before they take her back. I give the phone back to Tina and wipe the tear from my cheek. We drive in silence.

The scope of Mom's stomach reveals thirteen ulcers, one bleeding into her abdomen. She can die from this if we do nothing.

What now? She is still sedated, tucked away in her room, while Tina and I make our way down the hall to an empty waiting area. We settle into a corner, quiet and tense. "What do we do?" I whisper. "Do they operate? Is this the end? If we do nothing, she'll bleed out."

We stare at each other, speechless. No words, just tears. We knew this moment was coming, but knowing doesn't make deciding any easier. Do we intervene? Do we let nature take its course? Neither of us wants to be the one to choose.

Two middle-aged women—decisive, stubborn, and more like our mother than we care to admit—make the only logical decision: we'll call our sons. They'll know what to do. Mine's an EMT and firefighter, cut from the same cloth as my father. He'll know. Tina's son was the one who found her after the initial fall, after four days alone on the floor. He'll know too.

After hearing them out, we regroup. Their advice is simple, aligned, and somehow obvious: *Ask her what she wants.*

Of course. Sometimes the clearest minds aren't the oldest; they're simply the ones not paralyzed by fear, exhaustion, or the weight of history.

Mom's awake. Still capable of making decisions. So, we return to her room, stand by her bedside, and gently lay out the options. She listens, then answers without hesitation: "Well, of course they need to do the procedure. Why wouldn't they?"

Just like that, the fog lifts. The staff springs into motion, prepping for transfer to a Trauma One hospital equipped to handle the procedure. We're back in the game—because she said so.

They transport her at midnight. The surgeon is on tap to see her first thing in the morning. I follow the ambulance to the new hospital, meet the ICU nurse assigned to Mom's room, make sure her medications and allergies are noted in the chart, (a much too familiar routine) and head back to her house at 2 a.m. hoping to get a few hours of sleep before returning to the hospital.

The next three weeks pass in a haze. The surgery, by all clinical accounts, is a success. But Mom is never the same. She moans constantly, her body wracked with discomfort. Her mouth is dry. Her skin hurts. Bedsores have progressed to severe, open ulcers. She's agitated, restless, unreachable. After a few days, she is moved from the ICU to a regular room, but nothing soothes her. Tina and I try everything—music, conversation, silence. Still, she cries out, eyes closed, voice strained: "Help, help."

"The nurse is right here. How can we help?"

"I don't know," she whispers. "It just hurts."

I return day after day, sitting by her bedside, praying for a shift, a moment of peace. But it never comes. The moaning continues. The pleading doesn't stop. There's no comfort—for her, or for me.

The Key Phrase That Opens the Door to Hospice

Hospital time moves differently—days blur, stretch, and collapse into each other. What feels like a few moments becomes a week. Dr. Stephenson, the attending physician since Mom's transfer from the ICU, has been monitoring her decline. After days of moaning, groaning, and pleading for help, he finally broaches the subject we've been waiting for: hospice.

Yes! Finally, a doctor who acknowledges that she's not improving. She's in chronic pain. The internal bleeding has stopped, but she's miserable. And while death may not be immediate, it is imminent. And there it is. These magic words—death is imminent—unlock the path to hospice care.

"The hospital staff can help you get started," Dr. Stephenson offers gently. I thank him, but decline. We've already arranged hospice care, anticipating this moment long before it arrived.

Hospitals often have dedicated hospice wings where comfort care is provided, but she won't be staying here. She will return to the nursing home—where the staff knows her, where her friends are. Despite her years of stubborn resistance, the long-term care facility has become her home. She feels safe there. She feels loved there. And the people who care for her, day in and day out, have become more than caregivers. They are family.

Have a plan and decide if you want to use a hospital-initiated hospice service provider, or whether you want to find your own hospice company. Since hospice is a Medicare covered service with state governed requirements, switching from one provider to another can be messy.

For a patient to be admitted and authorized for hospice care, they must meet specific criteria. According to *Criteria for Determining Hospice Appropriateness - Hennepin Healthcare*, the patient should meet the following criteria:

- Life limiting condition

- Patient/family informed of the condition

- Patient/family has elected palliative care

- Clinical progression of the disease is evidenced by one or more of the following:
  - » Serial physician assessment
  - » Laboratory studies
  - » Radiologic or other studies
  - » Multiple ER visits
  - » Inpatient hospitalizations

- Recent decline in functional status as evidenced by [the criteria listed].

  Karnofsky Status ≤ 50%
  - » 50% Requires considerable assistance and frequent medical care

  - » 40% Disabled; requires special care and assistance; unable to care for self; disease may be progressing rapidly

  - » 30% Severely disabled although death is not imminent

  - » 20% Very sick; active supportive treatment is necessary

  - » 10% Moribund; fatal processes progressing rapidly

- Dependence in 3 of 6 ADLs
  - » Bathing
  - » Dressing
  - » Feeding
  - » Transfers
  - » Continence of urine and stool
  - » Ambulation to bathroom

- Recent impaired nutritional status is evidenced by:

  Unintentional, progressive weight loss of 10 percent over the past six months

Meeting the Hospice Intake Coordinator

With Dr. Stephenson's guidance, I reach out to Alisha, the intake coordinator for the hospice company we've chosen—a recommendation from my friend Robin, who's become my rock throughout this caregiving journey. Though our mothers' paths differ in diagnosis and timeline, the emotional terrain—grief, worry, and the constant unknown—is something both Robin and I know intimately.

I send a text to Alisha late Thursday night. Dr. Stephenson is guiding us, but Mom's discharge is fast approaching, and decisions need to be made. Alisha—an experienced critical care nurse—understands the urgency. Even though it's her day off, she agrees to meet Tina and me the next morning.

We gather at the kitchen table, and Alisha begins to walk us through what hospice care truly means. She's warm, articulate, grounded, and sharp—someone who radiates both competence and compassion. I trust her instantly. Tina, ever cautious, remains reserved. But for me, this is the kind of guidance I've been craving: someone who can demystify the dying process, help me understand what is happening, what Mom is experiencing and prepare us for what lies ahead.

Alisha explains that hospice care supports not just the patient's physical comfort, but also their emotional and spiritual well-being—and that of the family. One of its core principles is honoring the individuality of faith, recognizing that not every patient or loved one shares the same beliefs. There's no assumption, no agenda, just presence and respect.

They navigate this fragile terrain with grace and clarity. And in this moment, I know they're exactly the kind of support I need to walk through this final chapter.

Tina, by contrast, is skeptical. She meets Alisha's warmth with resistance; her questions edged with defensiveness. I find myself wondering—who is Tina fighting? What fear is driving her pushback? Alisha is here to help. She's on our side.

Later, in private, Alisha offers insight: Tina needs something different. She's not looking for emotional reassurance—she needs data, science, clinical clarity. I'm seeking an expert in death, someone who can guide me through this unfamiliar terrain with compassion and precision. Tina wants proof. I want peace. And together, we're trying to act in Mom's best interest, making decisions she can't—or won't—make herself, just as we've done throughout this long caregiving journey.

Alisha answers every one of Tina's questions with patience and precision. Tina remains hesitant, but she doesn't stand in the way. To help her feel engaged, to give her a sense of ownership, I insist she sign all the hospice paperwork—and there's plenty. Mom named us both as co-medical power of attorneys in her trust, equal in authority. But when it comes to taking the lead, someone has to step forward. Tina is the eldest, and in this moment, it makes sense for her to be the one to sign.

Two hours later, it's done. Alisha has the signed medical power of attorney and the stack of legal documents needed to initiate hospice care. Finally, everything is in motion. Mom is officially under hospice care, and she'll receive the palliative support she deserves—care I can't provide, no matter how much I love her.

I've never witnessed someone dying. I don't know what it looks like, how close she is, or what signs to watch for. But the hospice team does. They've walked this path with countless families. Now they'll walk it with us.

Alisha assures us she'll take it from here. She'll complete the assessment at the hospital, determine what equipment needs to be in place for her return to the nursing home, and coordinate across all fronts—hospital staff, nursing home staff, hospital physician, nursing home doctor, and now her hospice physician.

Once hospice services begin, the hospice team becomes the central decision-makers. Orders, prescriptions, and care directives flow through them. They collaborate with both the hospital and nursing home teams to understand the entire medical, emotional, and psychological history. But from this point forward, hospice leads the charge guiding us through this end-of-life process.

As defined by the Centers of Medicare and Medicaid Services (www.cms. gov), "Hospice is a public agency or private organization or a subdivision of either that is primarily engaged in providing care to terminally ill individuals, meets the conditions of participation for hospices, and has a valid Medicare provider agreement."

Hospice care is an approach to caring for terminally ill individuals that stresses palliative care (relief of pain and uncomfortable symptoms), as opposed to curative care. In addition to meeting the patient's medical needs, hospice care addresses the physical, psychosocial, and spiritual needs of the patient, as well as the psychosocial needs of the patient's family/caregiver."

When hospice care begins, you may choose to bring your aging parent back to the comfort of home. Unlike in a long-term care facility where staff provide daily support, at home the family steps into those roles—bathing, changing, feeding, and managing medications.

Take time to research what hospice care truly entails—how it works, what services are offered, and how it supports both patients and families. Look into volunteer coalitions and state-specific organizations; many offer excellent resources to help in understanding the structure and philosophy behind hospice.

Even if a loved one isn't ready or eligible yet, it's wise to be prepared. Consider reaching out to a hospice provider for an informational interview. Ask questions. Learn the language.

It's especially important to understand how hospice care intersects with Medicare and Medicaid, and how the hospice team collaborates (or sometimes, takes over as the lead) with the existing medical team. This knowledge will empower effective advocacy in making informed decisions when the time comes.

Hospice can offer pain relief, comfort and support to patients and their families wherever the patient lives. Services that the hospice team provides include:

- Manages both the patient's pain and other non-pain symptoms
- Provides emotional support
- Provides needed medications, medical supplies and equipment
- Coaches family caretakers on how to care for their loved ones
- Provides family caregivers with needed time away from responsibilities (respite time)
- Delivers special services like speech and physical therapy when needed
- Provides short-term inpatient care when pain or symptoms become too difficult to manage at home

- Provides grief support to surviving loved ones and friends. Support can include conversations with the person and family members, teaching caregiving skills, prayer and phone calls to loved ones, including family members who live at a distance and companionship and help from volunteers

Clarifying Hospice: What It Offers—and What It Doesn't

Understanding what hospice services do and don't provide helps with setting expectations in knowing what additional support or resources may be needed. Here are a few examples of what hospice services and Medicare do and don't cover at the time of this publication:

- The Medicare Hospice Benefit covers services, medications, supplies, and equipment that are related to life-limiting illness. It does not, however, cover expenses associated with room and board, <u>Who Pays for Hospice? | Medicare Coverage | VITAS Healthcare</u>

- Some may think hospice provides 24 hours a day, 7 days a week custodial care, or full-time care at home or at an outside facility. This is rarely the case. Although hospice provides a lot of support, most of the day-to-day care of a person dying is provided by family and friends. <u>Frequently Asked Questions About Hospice Care | National Institute on Aging (nih.gov)</u>

- A hospice team or registered nurse is often available by telephone 24 hours a day, 7 days a week, even on holidays and weekends.

- Along with medical decisions, hospice teams can also help the dying feel a sense of control by discussing their wishes – What type of funeral do they want? Are there specific songs or flowers they would like? What are their wishes for their estate?

After a loved one passes, hospice continues to support families through free bereavement services, including grief counseling, support groups, memorial activities, and practical guidance. These services typically last for up to thirteen months after death, ensuring families are not left alone in their grieving process.

CHAPTER 21

Mom is Dying

Topics

— What the Body Tells Us:
Indicators of Approaching Death

— End-of-Life Meds

— Her Final Playlist: When Irish Eyes Are Smiling
and Sweet Caroline

Some days I wish I could sit beside Mom for hours, just holding her hand. But I know that is more fantasy than reality. Even twenty minutes at her side has me scrolling social media and mindlessly unwrapping one Hershey kiss after another until a pile of silver wrappers fills the nightstand.

There is often an emotional complexity between an adult child caregiver and a dying parent—an ache that carries the imprint of old wounds and, at times, a longing for resolution. Not every relationship reaches forgiveness or closure; some goodbyes remain unfinished. This can complicate the realities of end-of-life care when we have no choice but to accept the inevitable truth: we can only make them comfortable and wait. Understanding hospice services and the physical signs of approaching death, can help families begin to prepare themselves in heart and mind for what's ahead.

What the Body Tells Us: Indicators of Approaching Death

It's week three of Mom's latest and final hospital stay. Watching her suffer is agonizing. She is rapidly declining. She's struggling to swallow. She's no longer carrying on conversations. Her eyes are closed all the time, and she cries out for help over and over again. Nothing brings her comfort. *How can I help take her mind off her pain?* I launch my playlist of Christian music and pray over her. My evangelizing just causes her agitation. I try a different approach, sharing stories about what the kids are doing. She listens briefly and resumes her wailing and cries. I summon prayer warriors from St. Louis to Texas, asking for prayers that she relinquish her fears and trust; that she finds peace. I feel as if she might die in the next couple of days. I'm unsure if she'll make it back to the nursing home and begin hospice care. Her vitals are plummeting. Her heart rate is slowing. Her blood pressure is low. *Maybe this is it. Maybe she's about to pass. Maybe this is what dying looks like.*

I've been at her bedside for hours. Listening relentlessly to her inconsolable moaning. I must step away. I need a break. I need rest. It is long past the end of visiting hours. Before leaving the hospital, I kiss her, tell her I love her and brace myself that this may be the last time I see her alive. I'm numb, empty and sad. Tears travel down my cheeks as I walk in a fog down the hospital corridor toward the exit.

The next day, Tina calls from the hospital. "She's awake. Her eyes are open. She's eating applesauce and drinking," she says. *What? No! I thought she was dying. What's this? She's rallying. I should be grateful, but I'm not. I just want all of this to be over. I have nothing left to give.* The flurry of emotions is maddening. I'm exhausted, disappointed, confused, and overwhelmed. I feel guilty and sad, angry and empty. Numb and lightheaded, I once again head back to the hospital. She's lived to fight another day.

Released from the Hospital

We're told they will release her in the next day or two. The doctor has ordered hospice services, explaining, "There's nothing more we can do for her." Death is imminent. It may not come immediately, but her time is drawing near.

The hospital social worker, hospice coordinator, and discharge nurse are all busy getting Mom ready to go. A private ambulance arrives and the medics transfer her from the hospital bed to the stretcher. She is heading back to the long-term care facility where things are familiar, where her house plants need watering, and grandkid pictures hang on the wall. Back to being with her family. Not Tina and me, but the family she lives with every day. The residents, nurses and care partners anxiously await her return. I know they take good care of Mom there, but when I see the outpouring of love as she's wheeled through the door, I have no doubt she is home, wrapped in love.

What Am I Looking For?

As Mom settles back in her room, hospice care begins. Her decline is undeniable. I've seen this coming—months, weeks, years in the making—and yet arriving at this threshold feels surreal. She's entering her final chapter, and I'm deeply grateful for the hospice team. They're not just here for her; they're here for me, too, helping guide me through the fog of what will happen next.

Hospice teams witness death every day. It's their world, guiding families through the final transition with clarity and care. But this is uncharted territory for me. I don't know what dying looks like. *What happens? How long does it take?* I crave concrete answers: the physiology, the signs, the timeline.

Until now, most people I've asked—nursing home staff, friends, social workers—have sidestepped the conversation, hoping to spare me. I appreciate the intention, but I need the truth. I want to understand what to watch for, the changes in behavior or body that signal the nearing end so I can be prepared. Hospice professionals know these answers, and I want, I need, their insight to bring shape to the unknown and help me feel less out of control.

I've never witnessed death before, and the uncertainty is unnerving. I don't know what I don't know.

She's in Good Hands

Now that Mom's new hospice-provided mattress and wheelchair are set up, I feel assured she is in good hands. I've been in Missouri for three weeks and I need to return home to Texas for the wedding of our best friends' son. I'm leaving her. Saying goodbye is difficult. I may never see her alive again and *I need to be okay with this.*

I am in Texas, But My Mind and Heart are in Missouri

Even though I'm hundreds of miles away, *how-is-Mom-doing* thoughts consume me. Dana, the hospice nurse, and I communicate via text a couple of times a day with an occasional phone call when texting doesn't suffice. It's Thursday. I've been home less than a week.

During one of our calls, Dana shares an interaction she's had with Mom who can't speak much. Dana says, "Your Mom said, 'I'm scared.' When I asked of what, Momma started crying."

She went on to explain the picture she painted for Mom in her mind, describing heaven as the best day of her life, only better.

"I asked Momma Marlene to think of a day when she felt beautiful, and happy, and loved, and safe–the most perfect day of her life. *That* is exactly what heaven was like. Joe is waiting for you there," Dana says.

Several years later, when Dana and I reconnected, she shared this story with me.

I distinctly remember Momma Marlene's anxiety and fear and how she melted into my arms when I—for the first time with one of my sweeties—wrapped her up, cradling her like a baby, holding her close, whispering in her ear, "We have everything under control. Your family will be okay if you let go, and Joe will be so excited to see you."

I had never "held" a patient before, but I wanted to surround her with warmth, comfort and safety. As she settled in, our bodies intertwined, I felt a sense of peace come over her, even if only for a moment until she needed another dose of comfort meds.

I can honestly say she was a patient that changed me. I typically hug and touch my sweeties, so they know they're not breakable, but cradling Marlene was different. It was angelic.

She continues, "She's getting close. I can't say exactly when she'll pass, but she's showing signs of transitioning. She's not eating. She's not drinking. Her speech is minimal and nonsensical. She can't identify exactly what hurts, but she's definitely in pain from her Kennedy ulcer."

A Kennedy ulcer, also known as a Kennedy terminal ulcer (KTU), is a dark sore that develops rapidly during the final stages of a person's life. These ulcers form as skin breaks down, a natural part of the dying process. Not everyone experiences these ulcers in their last days or hours, but they're not uncommon.

Find more information at: Kennedy Ulcers: Pictures, Symptoms, Causes, Diagnosis, and Treatment (healthline.com)

During one of our phone calls, I asked Dana about other physical signs of the dying process, aside from not eating, and she shared a list of things to watch for.

- Breathing pattern changes
- Low blood pressure
- Difficulty or inability to swallow
- Pain
- Ear pinning - when the earlobes shrink and retract back towards the skull
- Skin receding from the hands or feet
- Mottling

Mottling occurs when the heart can no longer pump blood effectively. The blood pressure slowly drops and blood flow throughout the body slows, causing one's extremities to feel cold to the touch. Mottled skin before death presents as a red or purple marbled appearance. It is most often first seen in the feet, but travels from there up the legs. (More information is available on hospice websites)

Dana gently suggests, "If you want to see her, now is the time to come home. If you are okay with having said your last goodbyes, then that's okay, too. It is up to you."

There is genuinely no guilt. Dana is sharing her professional opinion and reporting on Mom's condition. I respect her for this.

Even though I thought I made peace with her dying when I left, I'm conflicted. My husband understands me and says, "You'll regret it if you don't go see her." I'm empty inside. There is nothing more to give. Nothing more to say. What if this is like every other time when I would think *it's the end*, and she keeps on living? I have no more energy to fight or negotiate with my sister. More from habit than intention, I book my flight and head back to St. Louis the next morning.

End-of-Life Meds

Dana has upped Mom's comfort meds gradually since I've been gone. Over the past few days, she's increased her Ativan to keep her comfortable. Ativan is a common end-of-life drug that helps with anxiety, insomnia, agitation and shortness of breath. Since Mom struggles to swallow, Dana uses a liquid form, filling the syringe and squirting the blue fluid under her tongue. It must taste awful because each time Dana does this, Mom scrunches her nose and makes a sour face.

> Nurses and hospice team members can toss around names of medications with ease. Don't be afraid to ask what the meds do. Sometimes one medication is called several things based on whether it is a brand name or generic drug. According to the Samaritan Life Enhancing website common end-of-life drugs include:
>
> - **Acetaminophen** *(pronounced uh-SEE-tuh–MIN–uh–fin)*. Known by the brand name **Tylenol**, it is used to reduce fever and mild-to-moderate pain. Acetaminophen can be taken in a pill by mouth or via a rectal suppository.
>
> - **Lorazepam** *(lore-AY-zuh-pam)* reduces anxiety, agitation, shortness of breath, and insomnia. Commonly available under the brand name **Ativan** or Lorazepam Intensol, it comes in either a tablet or liquid and is taken

by mouth. Lorazepam is one of the most-prescribed hospice medications. It can be given alongside morphine (described below) if needed for comfort.

- **Haloperidol** *(hal-oh-PER-uh-dol)* helps reduce agitation and nausea. Known by the brand name **Haldol,** it also treats certain psychiatric conditions.

- **Morphine** *(MOR-feen)* helps relieve moderate-to-severe pain and shortness of breath. It is the preferred hospice medication for pain. And it can prevent further breathing difficulties by decreasing shortness of breath.

I arrive on the usual evening flight, and I drop in at the nursing home to see how Mom's doing. She seems to be sleeping when I arrive. Her eyes are closed, and she doesn't open them to acknowledge my presence. During one of our talks, Dana reminded me that hearing was one of the last senses to go, so even though Mom doesn't respond, I talk to her anyway. I tell her I'm here, and how beautiful she looks in her leopard-print nightgown. She's a skeleton. I'm afraid even a kiss will hurt or break her. I lean in, barely touching my lips to her cheek. I spend a few moments by her side, and then I say, "I love you, and I'll see you tomorrow."

Families often approach hospice medications with differing points of view. Here, a pharmacist offers her perspective as a medication dispenser.

Years ago, I worked in a pharmacy that dispensed the "hospice comfort box" to various hospice companies. Back then, I assumed hospice nurses arrived, stayed, and cared for the patient until the very end. When my own mother began hospice at home, I quickly learned that wasn't how it worked. Hospice provided the medications, the hospital bed, and the supplies. They supported us, but we were fully responsible for her day-to-day care and for giving her medications. Even as a pharmacist, it was stressful and emotional.

When a loved one chooses hospice at home, the family becomes the one administering end-of-life medications. It can feel overwhelming to manage drugs with wide dosage ranges and the option to give them frequently. Over the years,

I've talked with many family members who were hesitant—or even refused—to give morphine or Ativan because they feared overdosing or shortening their loved one's life.

What I want people to understand is that these medications are not intended to hasten death. They are given to relieve symptoms. Many patients experience anxiety, fear, or discomfort as they approach the end of life, and these medications help ease that burden. They keep your loved one calm, comfortable, and at peace.

Offering this comfort is an act of kindness and mercy. As you do your best to love and support your family member, know that using the medications as directed is part of that care. The comfort box truly can be a gift in those final days

Rebecca Kitowski, RPh

Her Final Playlist: When Irish Eyes Are Smiling and Sweet Caroline

The next day, Tina and I meet at the nursing home. Dana is there, fluffing Mom's pillow, clipping her hair back with a butterfly barrette, and chatting about how healthy Mom's new shamrock plant looks. Mom tries to respond, and Dana speaks for her. "Yes, I know you got that from your daughter on St. Patrick's Day. I love it. I have a purple shamrock plant."

I learned that gospel music doesn't bring her comfort, so I'm changing things up. I crank the sound on my phone and launch *Sweet Caroline*. Tina, Dana and I serenade Mom, belting out the *duh-duh-duh* for all the residents to hear.

Next up, Tina cues up *Irish Eyes Are Smiling*. We continue singing along; it's just the three of us now as Dana has left to care for another patient across town. After a few more Irish ballads, we tell Mom we are heading off to get breakfast. We assure her we'll be back later.

As we wrap up breakfast, Tina and I head our separate ways. I return to Mom's room around three. Dana is there again, administering the afternoon meds. Discreetly, she shares what she is watching for, signs that indicate Mom is nearing transition. She flips the sheet back and looks at Mom's feet. No curling or mottling. Her feet still have good color.

"Like I said," Dana comments, "We don't know exactly." She kisses Mom, and says, "Bye Miss Marlene. Enjoy your daughter. I'll see you tomorrow."

Dana leaves, and I pull my chair up to the bed. My shoulders are even with Mom's. She is propped up, resting peacefully. I slide the bedside table over and open my computer. The room is silent except for the oxygen tank, filling and deflating with each labored breath like a bellows stoking a fire.

I'm distracted for a while studying an Excel file of Mom's finances when I realize something is different. Something has changed. The room is quiet. There is stillness. Mom's not breathing. I watch her chest. It is no longer moving. I touch her chin to close her mouth, but it falls open again.

And just like that, she's gone. A quiet, simple, unceremonious death. Nothing scary. No drama. She was here, and now she's not.

Every situation is different. I was given the gift of being beside Mom as she took her last breath — something I'd prayed for over the many years of caring for her. But not everyone dies in the presence of family. Experts often say that some people seem to hold on until their loved ones leave the room, then slip away moments later.

I call Dana, and when she answers, I say, "I think Mom's gone." We talk for a few minutes more about what I need to do next, and when she can return. She is in transit to see another patient who she expects will die shortly. I reassure her that there is no rush.

"Take care of what you need to. I'll see you when you free up and can get back here," I say. I end the call, step into the hallway, and ask the care partner, Lauren, to summon the nurse. "I need her now," I say emphatically. Not wanting to alarm those gathered for afternoon bingo, I lean in and whisper, "I think she's gone."

I call my sister, my husband and my kids and relay the news. I'm not sad, at least not right now. More bewildered, maybe stunned, but peaceful.

As the hours, days and weeks pass and I relive Mom's last day, I'm grateful and blessed that I was beside her as she took her last breath. I could have been in Texas. I could have been on a plane, but I wasn't. I was by her side, doing something normal, working on my computer.

For years, I've been immersed in this caregiver role. It's been ten years since the initial fall, the four days she lay on the floor, to now, me sitting beside her as she took her last breath. And suddenly I realize my job here is done. I promised Dad before he died that I would take care of Mom, and I kept my promise.

The anxiousness, the uncertainty, the tension that wells up in my shoulders and the paralyzing jolt that shoots through my body every time I get a call from the nursing home, are over. I can exhale. I can breathe. Ironic. Mom's last breath gave me my first deep breath in a long time. I'm no longer scared. She's at peace, and now, so am I.

My 'project manager of Mom's life' role isn't complete just yet. There are still tasks to complete and phone calls to make, but the emotional toll of unpredictability is over.

CHAPTER 22

Mom Died, Now What?

Topics

— Immediate Steps After a Death:
Planning a Funeral or Celebration of Life

— So Many Decisions—No Time for Mourning Yet

— Balancing Emotion and Finances
When Funeral Planning

— Strategies for Covering Funeral Costs

— Setting Up an Estate Checking Account:
Managing Bills and Reimbursements

— Finalizing the Estate: Clearing the Home
and Preparing for Sale

She's gone. This expected, predictable end brings another flood of emotions. Relief, grief, sorrow, emptiness, and peace. As difficult as this journey has been, it is over in an instant. Life changes in an instant-*again*. I acclimate to the new role of "Project Manager of Mom's Life" and suddenly, I'm terminated. Fired. On one hand this comes as a welcome relief. On the other I come to the stark realization that Mom was the last connection to this city where I grew up. With nothing holding her back, Tina will be selling her house and moving closer to where her son lives. I no longer have a reason to return.

Immediate Steps After a Death: Planning a Funeral or Celebration of Life

Mom died, now what? The most immediate need following a death is dealing with the body. Since she died in her room at the nursing home and we have hospice services in place, they guide us on what to do next. The nursing home care partners ask if I want to be in the room while they clean her up. I decline. Instead, I step into the hallway call my sister, husband and sons. I send text messages to friends and relatives who are up to date on Mom's situation, those who know she's in hospice and that her passing could be any day. I'm not emotional. No tears, yet, just reporting on the news of the moment. I feel bewildered, almost like I'm in a fog. I'm not sure if it is shock or a sense of emptiness as her spirit is no longer a part of this earth.

Mom never talked about death, and she had no interest in making funeral arrangements. The only decision she made was that she wanted to be next to Dad in the columbarium (which Dad called 'the wall') at church. When he died, Mom purchased a niche where both their urns would be laid to rest. The plaque on the columbarium wall is already in place. It's just missing Mom's year of death, which we now know.

Although Mom avoided conversations about her own mortality and never made formal plans, she occasionally dropped hints. "I think we did a good job with your dad's celebration of life," she'd say. "I'd like something like that—lighthearted and uplifting."

Traditional funerals unsettled her. The rituals—visitation at the funeral home, pallbearers, casket processions, graveside ceremonies—felt suffocating. She attended only when absolutely necessary, often leaving shaken and anxious. The whole experience triggered her physically, sending her blood pressure soaring and edging her toward panic.

Honoring her in death as she lived her life, Tina and I set out to create an experience that is uniquely Mom. As often as Tina and I disagree and struggle with communication, ironically, planning the celebration of life is seamless. Instead of friends and family paying their respects at a mortuary, we opt to host an open house. Mom loved her home and all it represented, and celebrating her life where her door was always open and all were welcome makes perfect sense.

Before visitors arrive, the grandkids roll up their sleeves and head to

Lowe's for a load of mulch. Their mission? Spruce up Mardy's house for the party. They pull weeds, replenish the mulch beds, plant flowers and wash down the patio. What better way to honor their grandmother than to give back to her the gift of love through hard work? Refreshing her garden would have made her smile.

With her ashes in a shamrock-embossed urn perched on the living room sofa table, friends new and old, stop by to visit, drink a beer, eat a sandwich and gather in the kitchen. A slideshow commemorating her life plays on TV screens throughout the house, and the grandkids wager a friendly game of billiards in the basement.

Late afternoon, we all head to the church columbarium where our parents' godson, who is a church deacon, says a prayer. We lovingly tuck her urn into the wall niche, where she belongs, right beside Dad.

> An alternative to burial or cremation is body donation (also called *anatomical donation*). This is when a person chooses to donate their body after death for medical training, scientific study, or research. Medical schools, research institutions, and programs use donated bodies to teach anatomy, develop surgical techniques, and advance understanding of diseases.

So Many Decisions—No Time for Mourning Yet

There are many ways to lay a loved one to rest, from traditional burial to cremation to scattering ashes in a meaningful place. Each path carries its own set of choices and navigating them while grieving can be overwhelming.

If planning a funeral or celebration of life for the first time, it may be helpful to learn more about the role of a funeral director. These professionals coordinate every aspect of the service, including transporting the body to the funeral home and burial site, overseeing embalming and preparation, managing necessary paperwork, assisting with obituary writing, and guiding the family through each step with care and clarity.

Balancing emotional needs, financial realities, and the desire to honor someone's life is no small task. Thoughtful advance planning can ease the burden, offering clarity and reducing stress during an already difficult time.

This isn't an exhaustive list but some time sensitive decisions may include:

- **Transporting the Deceased**—When a person dies, the body must be transported somewhere. A body removal attendant, sometimes referred to as a mortuary transporter or a body transport specialist, handles the respectful and dignified handling and transportation of deceased individuals. After the family is notified of the person's passing, the next call is to the mortuary, where a transport specialist is dispatched. Regardless of next steps, cremation, embalming and burial or donation, the body must be transported from its current location. There are strict, specific laws and documentation that must be completed when a body is transported.

- **Visiting the Mortuary**—Set aside time to speak with a funeral director to review arrangements. One of the first decisions is whether the loved one will be cremated or buried. This choice will guide the selection of a casket and whether the viewing will be open or closed. Consider transportation needs as well. Will a hearse be required, and should transportation plans be made for family members attending the service?

- **Obituary**—Decide who will take the lead on crafting the obituary. This can be done in collaboration with the funeral director or written independently by a family member or close friend. Consider whether to follow a traditional format or share a more personal, narrative-style tribute that reflects the unique life and spirit of the deceased.

- **Obituary Posting**—Obituaries are often posted on the mortuary's website, making it easy for friends and family to share the link through social media. When deciding how to spread the word, consider the age of the deceased and the habits of their peers— some may prefer reading obituaries in the daily paper rather than online. While print publication is less common today, it remains meaningful for many older relatives and friends. Keep in mind that local papers may charge for posting the obituary, and it can be costly.

- **Church**—Determine whether a church service will be part of the memorial plans. If so, contact the church office to confirm availability and discuss logistics. Seating arrangements, speakers, and the creation of a printed program for the congregation may need to be addressed. Even in cases where the service isn't held at the church, coordination may still be necessary—such as arranging a graveside service or opening and closing the columbarium niche.

- **Eulogy**—who will deliver the eulogy? Will someone speak about the deceased?

- **Music**— Consider whether music will be part of the visitation or church service. Specific songs may be chosen to reflect the life or faith of the deceased. Decisions may include whether to invite someone to sing, use live musicians, or rely on those provided by the church. Thoughtful musical selections can offer comfort and connection. Remember, it is customary to offer financial compensation to musicians.

- **Flowers**—Consider whether floral arrangements will be placed near the casket or urn, and if so, what style or type feels appropriate.

- **Charity**—If the deceased had a favorite charity, donations in their honor may be a meaningful alternative to flowers. Contacting the organization in advance can help clarify how to direct contributions—some may offer a dedicated webpage or donation link.

- **Death Certificates**—The mortuary typically handles the ordering of death certificates, and it's wise to request more copies than expected. Investment accounts, bank accounts, sale of a house, insurance companies, automobile sale transactions, all want a copy of the death certificate. Some entities accept electronic versions, others require the original certificate with an embossed seal.

Balancing Emotion and Finances When Funeral Planning

A frequent area of conflict when dealing with the deceased is how much to spend on the funeral. If there are minimal funds available, you will need to make fiscally responsible decisions while honoring the deceased. This can be challenging. Inversely, if there are monies available, offspring may want to minimize funeral expenses to maximize their inheritance. Whether there is a lot of money or none, deciding what to spend on funeral expenses can be stressful. Research prices and set a budget ahead of time to help mitigate emotionally-charged decisions and ward off conflict.

Historically, price shopping for things such as caskets or urns, funeral flower sprays, and prayer cards wasn't an option. These fees and service offerings were offered up in 'pricing packages' by a funeral director. Today, online marketplaces offer transparent pricing for everything from headstones to memorial keepsakes. Custom printing websites also make it easy to design programs or prayer cards tailored to the occasion. Deciding which tasks to handle personally versus those to delegate to the mortuary team often depends on available time, budget, and comfort with DIY projects. Some may choose to create a memorial slideshow, while others prefer handing over a stack of pictures and having the mortuary director take care of it.

Funding Funeral and Burial Costs

As much as I think I have my act together related to managing finances over the past several years, I am still surprised in the end. In spite of my organization and tracking on Excel spreadsheets we are caught off guard.

The week Mom was released from the hospital into hospice care, I reviewed her investments and opted to cash out her Individual Retirement Accounts (IRAs). Understand that I am not providing financial guidance. Contact a financial advisor for advice. In our situation, cashing out Mom's IRAs and having the account taxed at her tax bracket made sense. Along with moving monies, I also confirmed that beneficiaries were in place, so there were no complications. To my surprise, I discovered that neither my sister nor I was authorized to sign on her checking account. There were no beneficiaries listed.

This was a problem because I knew that the moment she died, no one would have access to funds in the account and the account would go into probate. The morning before Mom died, I headed to the bank with the power of attorney document and her living trust in hand. There was a glitch. Since no beneficiaries were designated and no other signers were on the account, I couldn't add myself. I couldn't add my sister.

Even if online access to financial accounts is available after a person's death, don't take action. Any activity, such as logging in or moving funds after the official time of death, can raise red flags. Financial institutions may interpret this as a potential security breach, triggering reviews by legal, cybersecurity, or compliance teams. What might seem like a simple online inquiry can quickly escalate into a formal investigation, adding unnecessary complexity to an already difficult time.

The bank advisor recommended adding the living trust as the beneficiary of the account, but it was Saturday and the bank's legal department was closed. I had to wait until Monday. I was stuck, and Mom died that evening. The moment she passed, her checking account and savings account were frozen.

If financial power of attorney on accounts has not been invoked prior to the person passing, exhale and slow down. The self-service process of managing things online has closed. From this point forward, coordination must happen directly with financial institutions. This means booking appointments, explaining the circumstances to representatives, and setting up recipient or trustee accounts. The takeaway message: the process is slow, the steps are numerous, and personal control has shifted. What once felt manageable now requires outside coordination and patience.

Strategies for Covering Funeral Costs

Since neither my sister nor I are listed on Mom's checking account, we can't access funds. The account is frozen. The moment she died, the rules change, and we need to figure out how to deal with final expenses, including funeral services, medical bills, and household utilities. I didn't see this coming. I had assumed we could use the inheritance funds to pay for funeral expenses, but no, that's not how it works. Anyone not listed as a signer on a checking account is responsible for paying costs upfront. And this is exactly what Tina and I had to do.

Realizing that funeral costs need to be covered out-of-pocket and reimbursed later by the estate, we keep meticulous records—saving receipts and logging every expense in a shared spreadsheet file. What starts as a simple expense tracking worksheet quickly expands into a multi-tab workbook with funeral planning activities, to-do lists, and a project plan for closing the estate. Here are the things we track.

Tab 1—Funeral To-Do List

> Gather pictures, scan them and create a slideshow
>
> Order catering
>
> Inform work of bereavement leave
>
> Drop off donation check to the church
>
> Order prayer cards and flowers
>
> Deliver clothes to mortuary
>
> Write obituary

Tab 2—Gifts and Donations

> This multi-column tab is for keeping track of names and addresses of gifts, donations made to charities, and condolence messages. This is for thank-you note tracking. It is easy to forget the fresh pan of brownies the neighbor drops off unless it's recorded.

Tab 3—Expenses

> Some expenses are charged to Tina's credit card and some to mine. We document who is paying for what so we can

reimburse ourselves when the estate accounts are unfrozen. Money management can cause conflict even in the most congenial relationships, and if siblings don't get along, it can become a flash point. Tina and I handle this part well. We each record what we spend for reimbursement when funds are available.

Sections on this tab include:

Funeral Expenses

Garage Sale/Estate Sale Income and Expenses

Household Expenses

Investment Account Inheritance

Medical Expenses

Tab 4—Antiques

This list includes antiques and heirlooms that require research to assess their value.

Tab 5—Project Plan

Along with tracking expenses, we also add a project plan worksheet to the file. The role of managing affairs doesn't end with her passing. There's still a long list of responsibilities involved in settling the estate. The project plan outlines specific tasks within each category, along with key milestones, including:

Funeral Coordination

Legal

Finances

Listing and Closing House Sale

Prepping for House Clean Out

Garage/Estate Sale Readiness

House Closing

Selling Mini Van

Even if the funeral arrangements are prepaid, have a plan. Choose to have a surviving beneficiary added to the checking account in advance or set aside funds allocated to survivors ahead of time to cover expenses until inheritance funds become available.

MEETING WITH THE ATTORNEY FOR THE LIVING TRUST

I contact the estate attorney, notifying him of Mom's death and asking about next steps. The receptionist offers condolences and reassures me with a touch of humor. "It's not like collectors can ruin her credit rating," she says. "We can schedule time for you to meet with Mike in six weeks."

Six weeks! I need to talk to him now. The urgency I feel doesn't match the pace of the legal process. Once again, I'm face-to-face with a lesson in patience, one I struggled to master throughout Mom's healthcare journey. As much as I want to move quickly and tie up loose ends, I have no choice but to wait my turn and follow the lawyer's timeline.

When the appointment finally arrives, the meeting is productive, but not in the way I'd hoped for. My eagerness to hurry things along is met with a reminder that estate matters take time, and resolution may be months away.

The attorney, once warm and accommodating during the creation of the living trust, now comes across as more dismissive. Perhaps it's because Tina and I have done our homework, arriving with pointed, well-informed questions. We can manage many tasks ourselves, but a few items require his expertise. And with each request for assistance, his compensation increases.

After reviewing the trust and assessing what's needed, Tina and I identify three areas where legal support is essential:

- **Drafting the Letter of Trust**—This formally transfers executor authority from Mom to Tina and me, allowing us to act on her behalf and carry out the instructions outlined in the trust. This step is crucial for moving forward, as the power of attorney that governed financial decisions during her life became invalid upon her death.

- **Securing a Tax Identification Number for the Estate**—Since Mom's social security number is no longer valid, this new identifier is necessary to handle financial matters on behalf of the estate. It enables the opening of a dedicated bank account to pay bills, reimburse out-of-pocket expenses, and deposit incoming funds such as a nursing home refund, a medical premium reimbursement, and an income tax refund check.

- **Filing Probate Documents**—Because Mom's checking account is now frozen and no beneficiaries were named, we need the estate attorney to file the necessary paperwork with the probate court to authorize access to those funds.

WHAT IS PROBATE?

With the accounts locked and no access granted to either my sister or me, the next step is submitting accounts without a designated beneficiary and ad hoc checks that arrive made payable to Mom, to probate. Simply mentioning the word probate elicits groans—and for good reason. While filing with probate court isn't technically difficult, the process is slow and often stalled by a backlog of other clients the attorney is working with. What should be a straightforward submission—a document and justification for releasing funds to heirs—can take months.

When I ask, "What is probate court? Is there a hearing? Is attendance required? What happens after a ruling?" The attorney's response is surprisingly anticlimactic.

"It's not actually a court case. There's no appearance before a judge. It's simply a matter of submitting the case, and in return, a probate letter is issued authorizing heirs to access funds and act on behalf of the deceased." In layperson's terms, bureaucracy.

Setting Up an Estate Checking Account: Managing Bills and Reimbursements

Armed with the Letter of Trust, a new tax ID number, and Mom's death certificate, we are ready to open a checking account in the name of the trust. Finally, after two months, we can start the process of reimbursing ourselves and distributing inheritances to the grandkids.

The first bank we visit, where my husband and I have been customers for thirty years, proves to be frustrating and unproductive. Tina and I arrive for our scheduled appointment, armed with a three-ring binder containing Mom's living trust and all the documents we believe are required to set up a new account. But there's a snag: our parents' original trust was written twenty-five years ago. After Dad passed, Mom's updated trust incorporated the original, which means the bank now wants not only Mom's death certificate but Dad's as well.

Complicating matters further, there's no legal representative at the branch. The documents are scanned and uploaded for review, with a turnaround time of seven days. If anything is missing or the legal team requests additional information, the clock resets—another seven days before we can proceed. I remind the staff that I live out of state and only have five days left in town. I ask the acting branch manager to contact their legal team directly to confirm we've submitted everything needed. He tells me there's no way to reach them—communication is strictly via email. No phone number. No direct contact. I'm stunned. Tina stays calm while I lose my temper and walk out. We head to another branch, hoping the issue lies with that particular manager. It doesn't. The second branch gives us the same answer.

Time is running out. I'm down to four days.

We try a different bank, only to learn their legal review process also takes seven days. It's maddening. Finally, at the third bank, we find a certified representative onsite who can help. No scanning, no waiting, no unreachable legal team. He reviews our documents—the Letter of Trust, Mom's death certificate, Dad's death certificate, and our driver's licenses— and sets up the estate account on the spot. Persistence pays off.

Relief. One major hurdle cleared. Financial handcuffs on the estate funds are released, and we can move forward paying bills such as utilities and taxes for the home that is now part of the estate. Expenses we've shouldered over the past few months are now reimbursable. Progress at last.

Finalizing the Estate: Clearing the Home and Preparing for Sale

In the weeks following Mom's death, Tina and I begin the daunting task of clearing out her house to prepare it for sale. Some suggest hiring an estate sale team, often called estate liquidators, who handle everything once personal items are removed. It's a hands-off option: they sell what's left, and in return, offer a modest payout, allowing the family to skip the emotional labor of sorting through a lifetime of belongings, hosting a sale, making donations, and discarding what should've been tossed years ago.

We choose the hands-on route and quickly learn it's not for the faint of heart. Eight consecutive twelve-hour days, step counters logging 20,000 steps daily, and sheer physical exhaustion become our reality. We fill a thirty-foot dumpster, make endless trips to Goodwill, post unique furniture on the social media marketplace site, and transform the three-car garage into a treasure trove for bargain hunters.

Price garage sale items to move with nothing priced less than $1. Group or 'kit' items in small boxes, bags or baskets. For example, we had a small box of patriotic items—a few flags, a scarf, a blanket and beads—the entire box was $5. Another example: we stuffed all the gift bags and wrapping paper into a large gift bag and sold it for $5. Remember, the goal is to move the stuff, and buyers need to get a better deal than if they shopped at their local dollar mart. We sold a marble-top credenza and a leather recliner for $25 each.

Though we question along the way whether the effort was worth the return, our answer is a definite yes. Not because the proceeds make a dent in our kids' student loans, but because it's what Mom would have wanted. She cherished her belongings, and garage sales, and whether hosting sales or hunting for deals, she found joy in it all. Honoring her spirit made every step worth it.

> *Durable medical equipment like a shower chair, walker, cane,*
> *and shower grab bars may not be quick sellers at a garage sale.*
> *Check your local area for donation centers. We found a donation*
> *center associated with a church that accepts durable medical*
> *items. They assess the items, refurbish them, and they are free*
> *to veterans and those who show a need, while being a tax-*
> *deductible donation for us.*

CLOSING ON MOM'S HOUSE

Four months after Mom's death, I make one last trip to St. Louis to close on the sale of her home. The process is simple, as the new homeowners are a high school friend and her husband. A neighbor recommends a local realtor to draw up the papers and help us close the deal. Knowing the new owners is special and a gift not lost on me. Mom loved her home, and even though she could not spend her last days there, we vowed not to sell it until she passed–a commitment we were fortunate to honor.

Mom's home meant love, family, community, and connectedness. She felt safe there, and it represented her most treasured life accomplishments. And her legacy continues with the love and commitment of the new family who now lives in the house on Hollow Creek.

I'm blessed to have a front-row seat as I watch future memories being made — grandkids placing rocks in Marlene's garden, disintegrating concrete yard statues brushed, repainted and brought back to life, and opening night high school theater production bouquets assembled from Mom's rose bushes.

Alas, the weight of her passing settles in as I walk through her home one last time. This isn't just the closing of her chapter—it's a farewell to the city where I came of age. Though I haven't lived in St. Louis for thirty years, it has always been home. A place to reconnect with extended family, visit familiar neighbors, and share stories with old high school friends. But now, the rhythm of regular visits ends. My parents are gone. My sister is relocating. And the thread that once tied me here has broken. I may return from time to time, but the deep connection is permanently severed.

It is now up to Tina and me, as the living legacies, to bridge the past and future. We are responsible for holding the values, stories, and spirit of those who came before, shaping the future with the wisdom of the past.

RESOURCES:

When-Someone-Dies-Checklist_Nov-2017_interactive.pdf (hospicegiving.org)

Checklist for What to Do After Someone Dies (aarp.org)

What does a funeral director do? (the role of a funeral director) (yourfuneralchoice.com)

When We Know Better, We Do Better

Topics

— Fifty-Six Ain't Twenty-Six

— Practical Strategies We Can Start Implementing Today

— Staying On Top of Our Health –
Screenings and Examinations

— Aging Out of Wild Weekends

— Self-Care is an Act of Love

— Detailing Our Wishes Before Others Have to Guess

— Minimizing and Downsizing – Cleaning Out Our Stuff

When you first opened this book, maybe you were feeling overwhelmed. Maybe you were searching for clarity, comfort, or a way forward. Whatever brought you here, this moment is your invitation to act.

For me, one of the clearest takeaways is the desire to live differently for me, my spouse and my kids. Clearing out clutter, simplifying my home, letting go of what no longer serves isn't just tidying up. It's an act of love. A gift to those who will one day walk through my space and remember me, not for the things I held onto, but for the life I lived.

Fifty-Six Ain't Twenty-Six

"Have a plan; 56 ain't 26." This is a simple phrase, but a powerful message on a Facebook post from a retired St. Louis police officer in his late fifties drawing nearly 600 views and 300 comments. Along with being in public service, Cedric served in the military and now spends his days as a music journalist and respected musician.

Curious enough, the social media post that drew so much attention wasn't about music, crime, or vacation memories. It came from a hospital bed. Cedric's previous post was a video from Chicago's Lakefront Trail: clear blue water, golden morning light, and the quiet joy of a solo bike ride. The next morning, he's in the hospital, legs wrapped in inflatable cuffs to prevent blood clots— a stark contrast to the serenity of a bike ride.

What happened? Heat exhaustion and dehydration.

Following a twenty-four-hour observation period, he was released. Grateful, humbled, and newly converted into a hydration evangelist.

Cedric and I went to high school together. We stay loosely connected through social media with rare opportunities for live conversations. When I saw his post, something changed inside of me. I needed to talk to him. His words carried weight. He understands the need to *plan for the unexpected.*

It's a theme that runs throughout this book, and Cedric's story is a powerful reminder of why it matters.

Before diving into the recent episode that landed Cedric in the hospital, let's rewind the clock. A few months prior, Cedric had collapsed in his apartment. When he came to, he called 911, and the experience was a wake-up call. Here's how he describes the initial incident.

> I tripped over an area rug in the living room. I couldn't catch myself because the spinal stenosis (the narrowing of spaces within the spine, which puts pressure on the spinal cord and the nerves that travel through the spine) has weakened the signal that goes from my brain to my legs. I fell on my left hip. Fortunately, nothing was broken, however, the incident made me realize something frightening: I live alone. How was I going to call for help if something had been broken? Who

was going to tell the paramedics about my medical issues and allergies? I'd never thought about that before. Now it was all I could think about!

My pal Oliver (name changed for privacy), who has a set of my keys for emergencies, suggested I get a medic alert bracelet. I did so immediately. I also instituted a few standing rules when I'm at home:

1. Keep the front door unlocked (you have to get through two levels of security and know where I live to get in).

2. Always have my phone with me.

3. Have a *go-bag* ready for emergency trips or potential hospital visits.

Fast forward to my most recent dehydration while bike riding event, and I'm thinking that my plan is what saved me. I was so out of it after passing out from my heat exhaustion, I couldn't think straight or find the strength to call 911 for several minutes. When I finally could, the paramedics got to me with relative ease.

Fifty-six ain't 26. I'm finally coming to grips with that. You've got to plan ahead, regardless of how healthy you think you are. It just might save your life one day.

What captivates me about Cedric is his clarity. He knows we're not getting any younger, and he embraces that truth without fear or denial. He's not giving up. He's not retreating. He's living a full, joyful life. But he's also planning. Cedric has taken steps to ensure that if something goes wrong, others know how to help. That kind of foresight isn't just practical—it's generous. It's the mark of someone who understands that aging isn't about surrendering; it's about adapting with intention.

Practical Strategies We Can Start Implementing Today

During our conversation, Cedric offered clear, actionable steps, practical strategies we can start doing today.

WHAT WOULD YOU LIKE TO TELL PEOPLE ABOUT YOUR PLAN?

"I would hope that my incident helps others to do the same; face the facts. We are our parents. We can't pretend we aren't getting older. There's a difference between getting old and aging. Getting old is a mindset, and aging is what happens to you naturally. My time in the Air Force and my career as a cop trained me to anticipate and have a plan.

With my first fall, I was 12 feet away from my phone and 25 feet from the front door. I live alone. How was I going to get help? That was my wake-up call, and I realized I needed to get things in order.

I started my preparedness plan. I ordered a medical alert bracelet. I wear it all the time. I'm a diabetic, so my medical condition and emergency phone numbers are listed. Sometimes people take it off to shower. That's stupid. Don't do that. Most falls happen in the shower. Wear it all the time. You need first responders to know about you even if you can't communicate, and the medical alert bracelet tells them critical information.

The next thing I did was write a detailed letter. I gave a copy to Oliver, my emergency contact, and he and I went over it. He knows exactly what to do in the event of an emergency. The letter outlines what to do with my apartment, who to contact in St. Louis, and what to grab if I'm in the hospital. It's all in there. He also has a key to my apartment."

WHAT DETAILS ARE IN YOUR EMERGENCY LETTER?

"I document all the things that need to be turned off or checked if my apartment is empty. Check the stove; check to see if water is running; turn off the TV. I do this because if I passed out, you don't know what I could have been doing at the time, and if Oliver is in a hurry, which he likely is if this is an emergency, he might need a reminder of things to check to secure my apartment.

I don't have any pets, but if you do, include instructions on what to do with them. Minimally, feed the pets, empty the trash, and clean out the fridge.

You also need to document your list of medications. Make sure you keep your medications organized and in their original medicine bottles. Also, list any allergies you have.

I also have a to-go bag packed in my closet. I have clothes, underwear, a phone charger, toiletries, socks, a pair of shoes, the works. You should also include some cash. In the letter, I instruct Oliver to grab my to-go bag and bring it to the hospital. On my last test run, I discovered I was missing earbuds from my to-go bag. I've since added them."

Are There Other Details That You've Documented?

"I also have clear instructions about what to do if I lose consciousness. There is a complete list of people to call with their phone numbers. The letter explains that Oliver is to kick off a call chain to notify people. The key is to be ready."

Most of us know our own vital information, but in an emergency, it's not about what *we* know, it's about what others can access quickly. That's why it's essential to have important documents organized and readily available for your emergency contact or care team.

Consider including:

- Military discharge papers
- Cremation or burial preferences
- Trust or will documentation
- Property distribution instructions
- Access details for bank accounts and credit cards
- Contact information for legal counsel, if applicable

Having these materials in one place, clearly labeled and easy to find, can ease decision-making and reduce confusion."

What Advice Can You Offer When Someone Says I'm Not That Old Yet?

"We are all susceptible to falling just like anyone else. Health status is irrelevant. Something can happen at any point, and you need to be prepared."

If you live alone, consider consulting a legal professional to prepare documentation covering financial details such as bank accounts, investments, and credit cards. Including information such as login credentials is also helpful, and then store this information in a secure location, like a safe deposit box or with someone you trust implicitly.

Cedric's story, caring for aging parents—it all points to one thing: we are being called to act. One of the most profound lessons in the aging parent journey is a reminder to care for ourselves. Supporting an aging parent reveals, often painfully, what may lie ahead in our own lives. It's both a wake-up call and a roadmap. And once we've seen what's coming, we owe it to ourselves and those we love to respond with intention.

Here, I challenge each of us to reflect on our own destiny. There's no crystal ball to tell us when our health might falter or what challenges await. Yes, science and technology will continue to reshape what's possible, but doing nothing isn't an option–at least not a good one.

We must challenge ourselves to look ahead. Organizing personal details isn't just about being prepared; it's about making it easier for others to support us when we need them the most. I don't want my legacy to end with my children scrambling to figure things out. I want to leave them clarity, not confusion.

Staying On Top of Our Health – Screenings and Examinations

We need to take care of ourselves by staying on top of annual screenings and examinations.

Annual Physical—Ask questions, be honest with the physician about mental and physical health and bring up any changes since the last exam. If blood testing is done, inquire about the results.

Prescription Medication—Be diligent about taking prescribed medications and talk with the doctor if they no longer seem effective. Body chemistry changes over time, and adjustments to medications may be needed.

Preventive Screenings—Preventive care is about playing the long game. It's the quiet, consistent work of investing in future health. This means prioritizing screenings that catch problems early, before they become crises. No one looks forward to a colonoscopy, but it's one of the most effective tools we have for early detection. Women should make annual mammograms and gynecological exams a priority, and men need to stay on top of prostate health. If a specialist is recommended, don't wait. Get that appointment on the calendar. Taking action now means fewer regrets later.

Dermatology Exam—Sunlight offers a natural source of Vitamin D, but it also carries potential risks, particularly for individuals with a family history of skin cancer. Regular visits to a dermatologist and annual skin screenings are an essential part of preventive care. Early detection can be lifesaving, and a brief skin check represents a meaningful step toward long-term health and well-being.

Annual Hearing Exam—Another important screening is a hearing exam. Hearing loss often creeps in gradually, and many people delay addressing it. But recent research published in *JAMA Neurology* shows that treating hearing loss early, especially between the ages of sixty and seventy, can significantly reduce the risk of developing dementia later in life.

Using hearing aids isn't just about improving communication; it's about protecting the brain. The study found that individuals who addressed hearing loss earlier had notably lower rates of cognitive decline. By addressing hearing loss earlier, individuals may reduce this cognitive strain and preserve brain health. It's a powerful reminder that proactive care doesn't just improve quality of life—it may help preserve it.

To explore the full findings, visit Hearing Health & Technology Matters.

Annual Eye Exam—Just as annual hearing screenings are essential, regular eye exams deserve equal priority. Vision changes can be gradual and easy to overlook, but they carry serious consequences. Research shows that consistent eye care can significantly reduce the risk of falls, which remains one of the leading causes of injury-related deaths among adults over sixty-five.

Clear vision isn't just about seeing well, it's about moving safely, navigating confidently, and maintaining independence. Prioritizing eye health is a simple yet powerful way to protect both body and mind.

Aging Out of Wild Weekends

As we inch closer to retirement, it may be time to rethink lifestyle habits. An adult beverage on the weekends or when socializing with friends may be part of the fun in celebrating, but there may be a point to reconsider consumption levels.

ALCOHOL AND AGING—HIDDEN HAZARDS

Increased sensitivity—As we age, body composition changes. Less muscle mass and water content mean alcohol has a stronger effect. Even moderate drinking can lead to higher blood alcohol levels.

Fall risk—Alcohol impairs balance and coordination, increasing the likelihood of falls, which are a leading cause of injury-related death in adults over sixty-five.

Medication interactions—Older adults often take multiple medications, and alcohol can interfere with their effectiveness or cause dangerous side effects.

Mental health impact—Alcohol misuse in older adults is often underdiagnosed. It can worsen depression, anxiety, and cognitive decline.

Organ damage—Long-term drinking increases the risk of liver disease, heart problems, and certain cancers, even more so in aging bodies.

Similar to the effects of alcohol, smoking can exacerbate declining health.

SMOKING AND AGING—COMPOUNDING DAMAGE

Cognitive decline—A meta-analysis published in *BMJ Open* found that current smokers had significantly lower odds of healthy aging compared to never-smokers. Research shows that smoking increases the risk of Alzheimer's by about 30%, and smoking increases the risk of dementia, stroke, and vascular disease.

Respiratory issues—Aging lungs are less resilient. Smoking accelerates the decline in lung function and increases the risk of chronic obstructive pulmonary disease (COPD).

Cardiovascular strain—Smoking contributes to high blood pressure, atherosclerosis, and heart disease, conditions that become more dangerous with age.

Delayed healing and immune suppression: Older adults who smoke may experience slower recovery from illness or surgery and are more prone to infections.

Self-Care is an Act of Love

When I was growing up, my mom was a heavy smoker—multiple packs a day. But the moment her first grandson was born, she quit cold turkey. Determination and perseverance were her trademarks, and she carried those same qualities into her approach to food and health.

HEALTHY EATING

One of the most valuable life lessons she passed down was the importance of nourishing the body with purpose. Long before "power foods" became trendy among fitness coaches, Mom was living what science now affirms: eating well is a cornerstone of aging well.

Her plate was always colorful with fresh vegetables, whole grains, grilled meats and poultry. And she never skipped breakfast. It was her way of fueling the day, setting a tone of care and consistency.

As we age, our nutritional needs shift. Metabolism slows, muscle mass declines, and the body becomes more sensitive to deficiencies. Prioritizing nutrient-dense foods—like leafy greens, berries, lean proteins, and healthy fats—can help maintain energy, support brain health, and reduce inflammation.

Mom understood this intuitively. Her habits weren't trendy, they were timeless. And they remind me that aging well is about feeding the body what it truly needs to thrive.

STAYING ACTIVE

One of the most pivotal lessons I learned while walking alongside my mother through her aging journey was the profound importance of movement—specifically, maintaining muscle strength, balance, and coordination. Aging naturally brings a gradual loss of muscle mass, which can make everyday tasks more difficult and increase the risk of falls and injury.

Staying active means improving and maintaining good balance. Balance isn't just a physical skill. It's a safeguard. It's what allows someone to step confidently into the shower, navigate a curb, or reach for a book on a shelf without fear. And it's not something we can afford to take for granted. Activities like yoga, tai chi, and stretching routines help preserve flexibility and joint mobility, while also calming the nervous system and improving posture. Programs like Silver Sneakers, Pickleball, and gentle resistance training offer accessible ways to stay active and socially engaged.

Staying active is essential for maintaining hip health, especially for women. Research shows that women account for nearly 80% of all hip fractures, a statistic largely driven by the sharp drop in estrogen after menopause, which accelerates bone loss and increases fragility. Studies show that older women with low bone density are experiencing their first hip fracture earlier in life, with a growing number of first-time fractures occurring in their sixties.

Core strength is especially vital. It stabilizes the spine and supports mobility. As safely as possible, continuing to move and strengthen the body is one of the most powerful forms of self-care.

I saw this firsthand with my mother. As her health declined, she moved from using a cane to a walker and eventually became fully dependent on a wheelchair. The transition was swift and sobering. It taught me that inactivity accelerates decline, and that even small efforts to stay mobile can make a meaningful difference.

STAYING MENTALLY STRONG

Mental decline is a common concern among aging adults, but it's not inevitable. Brain health isn't just about diet and exercise, it's also about connection and stimulation. Socialization plays a critical role in maintaining mental acuity. Regular interaction with friends, family, or community groups helps reduce isolation, boost mood, and keep the brain actively engaged in conversation, memory, and emotional nuance.

Technology can also be a powerful ally. Thinking games like *Mahjong, Sudoku, Wordle,* or digital crossword puzzles offer daily mental workouts that challenge memory, strategy, and pattern recognition. Video calls, online classes, and virtual book clubs can keep older adults socially connected and mentally sharp.

The takeaway? Protecting brain health isn't a single action. It's a series of choices. Stay curious. Stay connected. Whether it's a brisk walk, a shared laugh, or a round of Mahjong, each moment of engagement is a step toward preserving the mind.

GETTING A GOOD NIGHT'S SLEEP

Establishing healthy sleep habits can make a difference, and when snoring becomes a nightly norm, it might be worth exploring a sleep study to uncover what's going on beneath the surface. Disrupted sleep, often characterized by snoring, can increase the risk of dementia by accelerating brain aging, impairing cognitive function, and contributing to harmful changes like amyloid plaque buildup. Conditions like obstructive sleep apnea (OSA), a common cause of snoring, are particularly linked to these negative effects.

ORGANIZING OUR FINANCES

One of the most caring and considerate acts we can offer those who love us is to organize our financial affairs before they're left to navigate a tangled mess. It's not just responsible, it's compassionate. Over a lifetime, we accumulate homes, vehicles, retirement savings, and personal treasures. Before it's too late, we owe it to ourselves and others to clearly document our wishes. A will or trust is a roadmap. Without it, those left behind may face needless confusion, conflict, and heartache.

We plan for vacations. We plan for retirement. We need to plan for the inevitable. This means sitting down with a financial planner or elder law attorney to determine what's right for our individual situation and putting it in writing.

Another essential step: make sure every account—retirement, checking, savings, credit cards—has a designated beneficiary. It's a simple action that allows loved ones to act on our behalf when we no longer can, protecting our assets and the people who will carry our legacy forward.

Along with organizing finances, regardless of whether a formal will or trust exists, it's essential to establish Power of Attorney (POA) for both financial and medical decisions. A Financial Power of Attorney, also known as a Durable Power of Attorney (DPOA), allows a trusted appointee to manage accounts, pay bills, and handle legal matters if you're unable to do so yourself. A Medical Power of Attorney (MPOA) ensures that someone can make timely healthcare decisions on your behalf, especially in moments when you can't speak for yourself.

Without these documents in place, loved ones may be forced to navigate costly, time-consuming court proceedings just to be appointed as guardian or conservator.

Detailing Our Wishes Before Others Have to Guess

We all assume we'll have more time. But the truth is, tomorrow isn't promised, and that's why having courageous conversations with a spouse, child, or close friend is so important. These conversations lift the burden of uncertainty. They eliminate guesswork in moments when clarity is most needed.

While writing this book, I spoke with friends and experts covering many topics. One friend shared insights about relocating her aging parents—a thoughtful, proactive move. Just months later, I visited her in the hospital. She was on life support, having suffered a massive stroke on the sidewalk in front of her beloved church. Her husband and four children spent twenty-one agonizing days at her bedside, praying, consulting with doctors, and searching for signs of brain activity.

Engaging in difficult conversations matters. It's important to speak openly with loved ones about care preferences in the event of a stroke, whether it's a minor episode or a life-altering event. Clarifying choices, like staying at home versus moving to a skilled nursing facility, can ease future decision-making and ensure care aligns with personal values.

Discuss what happens when driving is no longer safe. Will you rely on a senior transportation service, or will someone help you navigate Uber?

These aren't easy topics. But they're necessary. Because when we speak our wishes aloud, we give our loved ones the gift of clarity and the confidence to act with compassion.

PRE-ARRANGE FUNERAL OR LAST WISHES

Planning and financing funeral arrangements is one of the most compassionate steps we can take to ease the burden for survivors. Whether you prefer a traditional burial, cremation, or wish to donate your body to science, documenting your choices brings clarity and comfort to loved ones during an otherwise overwhelming time.

Recently, my husband and I took this step ourselves. We met with funeral home directors, toured cemeteries, and explored the differences between burial and cremation. We learned about vaults, visitation options, church services, catering, and even limousine escorts. What surprised us most was the cost. Depending on location and services, funerals and cemetery plots can be triple what you might expect.

Because we approached this process while healthy and emotionally grounded, we could make thoughtful, frugal decisions. We compared prices, negotiated options, and even discovered a resale website offering unused crypts and burial plots. In one case, a family's situation changed. Extended family moved away, and they no longer wanted the family burial plot purchased years ago. After a re-deeding process, we officially secured our final resting place.

When grief strikes, rational thinking is often clouded. Negotiating under stress is difficult, and decisions made in haste can be costly. Planning ahead allows for sound, informed, and cost-effective choices, taking the guesswork out when emotions are running high.

Minimizing and Downsizing – Cleaning Out Our Stuff

When my mother and mother-in-law passed—just four weeks apart—my husband and I, along with our siblings, found ourselves sorting through two fully furnished homes, each filled with decades of cherished possessions.

My mother-in-law had saved every birthday card, anniversary note, and graduation program. Her outdoor shed held twenty years' worth of farm business files. And her love of Christmas? It lived in a closet overflowing with Santas, snowmen, and bric-a-brac she'd collected over a lifetime.

My mom's house was no different. Cabinet after cabinet held mismatched drinking glasses, each missing one or two from the set. My sister and I stared at her sixty-year-old wedding dress, its lace yellowed and crumbling, unsure what to do with something so sentimental yet so fragile.

Here's the hard truth: don't leave your stuff for your kids, family, or friends to sort through. Start now. If your children don't want your fine china today, they probably won't want it later. And if you haven't decorated with your Snow Babies collection in years, chances are you don't like them anymore. Let it go.

Minimize. Clean. Reduce. Simplify. Not because your life is ending, but because your time and energy are better spent living, not storing. Letting go of what no longer serves you is a quiet act of love. It's a gift to those who will one day walk through your home and remember you—not for what you kept, but for how you lived.

Helping others help us is about planning ahead and letting go of our pride. Aging is inevitable, and denial only delays the support we may one day need. The most compassionate thing we can do for ourselves and those around us is to take ownership of our future.

When we know better, we have a responsibility to act. Preparation isn't just practical; it's compassion for those who will care for us.

Since We Know Better, We Must Do Better.

www.ingramcontent.com/pod-product-compliance
Lightning Source LLC
Chambersburg PA
CBHW070611170726
48004CB00017B/90